One by One

Working with Dyslexia

The Story of
Dunnabeck and Kildonan

by
Diana Hanbury King

©2005

First Edition: May 2005

Designed and produced by
Rooney Design Group, Amenia, NY

ISBN 097672070-1

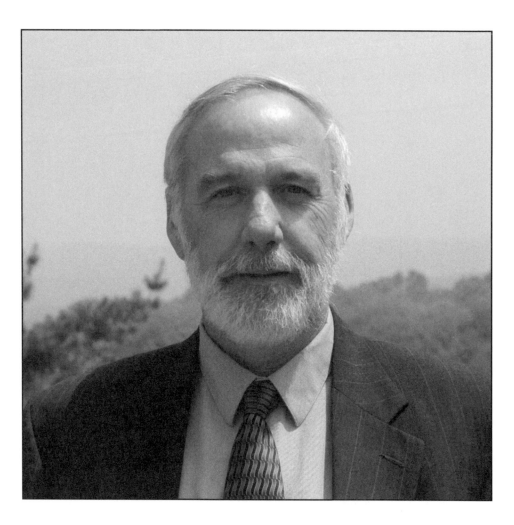

For Ron Wilson, headmaster of many years,
who has made into a permanent and wonderful institution
what I was only able to begin, with my heartfelt
admiration and gratitude.

I am deeply grateful to Dr. Robert Lane and to William Van Cleave for their invaluable editorial help, and to my sister, Jillian Poole, for her suggestions and encouragement.
-DHK

❧ Foreword ❧

I have been teaching dyslexic students all my working life. This book is an account of my experiences, and of the thousands of teachers and students with whom it has been my privilege to work. While the students remain the same—endlessly fascinating in their ways of learning and failing to learn—other things have changed during the past sixty years. There is less denial of dyslexia in the world as a whole. New technology makes the task of writing and reading easier. Technology has also enabled researchers to take a closer look at the dyslexic brain and to see differences that can no longer be denied. Finally, the importance of phonological awareness and of early intervention has been established.

Dr. Samuel Torrey Orton (1879-1948) was among the first to realize that dyslexia was the result of brain differences, rather than the emotional or sociological problems to which it had previously been attributed. Because he began work after World War I, he had the opportunity to dissect the brains of patients who had, as a result of wounds, suffered loss of the ability to speak, to read, or to write. By the time of his death, he had examined more brains than any other physician then living. Thus he was able to begin to localize those areas of the brain involved in language. Moreover, Dr. Orton realized that dyslexia was more than a reading difficulty; he titled his book *Reading, Writing, and Speech Problems in Children*. He worked with Anna Gillingham (1878-1948), a psychologist and gifted teacher, to devise effective teaching methods for these children. Unfortunately, the work of these two pioneers was largely unread and unrecognized by those in the teaching profession who were in a position to make the necessary educational reforms, and understanding of dyslexia was slow to spread.

Dyslexia, we now know, affects close to twenty percent of the population, equally distributed between male and female, but it was long believed to be a rare condition, affecting no more than two or three percent of the population, and at that mostly males. Those who could not succeed in school were tested, and when they were found to be intelligent their failure to learn was attributed to laziness or lack of motivation. Parents and teachers treated them accordingly, and when, not surprisingly, some of them developed emotional or behavioral problems, psychiatrists sometimes spent years trying to unravel the causes of their failure. Schools often claimed to recognize the existence of dyslexia, but would deny having any such students in their population. Recently, prominent individuals including Cher, Tom Cruise, Charles Schwab, and Henry Winkler have made a point of publicizing their own dyslexia, so that the label of dyslexia is less likely to be viewed as a unique disgrace. Nevertheless, this knowledge is still far from widespread in this country, and elsewhere in the world students are even more likely to go undiagnosed and untreated. This situation is a tragedy.

Technology is wonderful. A computer or laptop equipped with a spell checker and a grammar checker is a godsend to many dyslexics, and is often the one thing that will enable them to succeed in college, or in some cases to finish high school. Books on tape or CD may enable students to listen to all the Harry Potter books long before they can decode them. The technology for scanning texts and for speech-to-print—the latest miracle—continues to improve. But there is a catch. Schools are prone to provide students with tapes instead of teaching them to read. Young children who have difficulty with handwriting are encouraged to use computers rather than being given appropriate instruction. I was once called as an expert witness in the legal case of a tenth grader whose parents were in litigation with their school district. A virtual non-reader, he had every accommodation available, and his mother was spending her evenings helping him to cope with his assignments. Not surprisingly, he was getting good grades. The position of the school was that they were under no obligation to teach him to read and write. Of course, I took a different view. The school hearing officer sided with the school, but the parents appealed the matter, and the judge said I was right. He began to receive appropriate instruction and, within a year, he was reading at a high-school level and spelling at a seventh-grade level. Obviously, for a school system, it is cheaper to provide technology than to train teachers. But did you ever try to learn a foreign language from tapes?

The most exciting development in recent years has been our ability to watch the brain at work through magnetic resonance imaging (MRI). No longer do we have to wait until a person dies to examine a dyslexic brain—as did Dr. Orton. Scientists can watch the brain as it performs various tasks. The pattern of a dyslexic brain at work differs from that of an efficient reader. Even more miraculously, as we teach, using all the Orton-Gillingham strategies to activate new pathways among the neurons, the brain changes, becoming more like that of a normal reader.

Years ago, I was at a cocktail party when David Malin, then head of Jemicy School in Baltimore, said to me, "Doctor Compton has a son who cannot read, but he is sixteen, and of course it is too late...." Well, it certainly was not, and last I heard from Peter Compton, he had received a master's degree and was working as a social worker. Public school systems tend to provide little or no help beyond elementary school. Admittedly, it is more difficult to find the time for remediation when a student has to accumulate the necessary credits for graduation. But if students are simply passed along without receiving special help, they graduate unable to read or write.

Actually, there are advantages to working with adolescents. The reversals and confusions that plague younger students are more manageable. They are able to concentrate for longer periods of time and more readily grasp the rules and generalizations that govern the language. And, if we can succeed in motivating them, they will work tirelessly.

It is only in recent years that the importance of early intervention has been recognized. Phonemic awareness—the ability to discern the different sounds, or phonemes, that make up a word—is now widely accepted as a critical component in learning to read and write. But it has not always been so. As late as 1996 parents involved in litigation called me as an expert witness at a hearing in which the school had brought in a professor from Temple University as their witness. As he testified, I became upset at the extent of his ignorance. When he finished speaking, the parents' attorney leaned over and whispered, "Anything you would like me to ask him?" I said, "Ask him to talk about phonemic awareness." The professor, who incidentally was in charge of teacher training, hesitated, and said, "I am afraid that is not my field." The attorney then asked him to define the term, but he could not.

Beginning to train children in phonemic awareness before they enter first grade has proved to make a critical difference in learning to read. At-risk kindergarteners have been shown to catch up with their peers when provided with no more than a couple of months of teaching. There are now plenty of attractive games and materials available that make phonemic awareness easy to teach and fun for young children to learn. Certainly, by the time a child is five years old, and often sooner, after talking to parents and spending no more than half an hour with a child, a qualified person should have a pretty good idea as to a child's learning style and the likelihood of success in first grade.

Without appropriate intervention, children who are behind in primary school will continue to lag behind their peers at the end of high school and beyond. The non-reading third grader is at risk for life-long illiteracy. The high school student who cannot write is likely to drop out of school. Worst of all, dyslexic students who fail to master reading and writing grow up feeling stupid. It has been said, "Dyslexia will not kill you but it can certainly ruin your life."

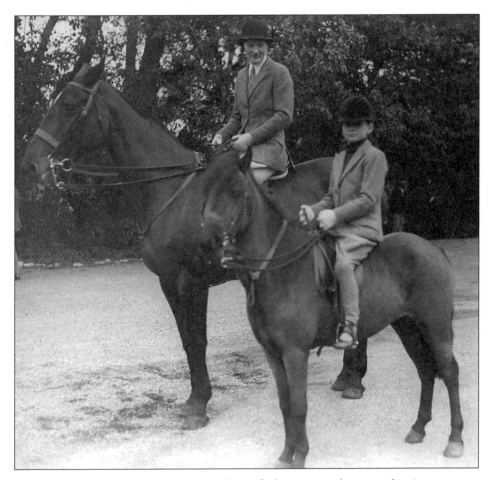

Taken in October 1935 when I was 8. I am foxhunting with my mother in Aldershot.

~ I ~

Growing Up

My sister Jillian and I grew up in England in rural Hampshire. Derbyfields, our country home, was a long pink cottage surrounded by flower and vegetable gardens and an apple orchard. In one corner of the orchard was a gate that led to the stables and the pasture. I was standing by that gate when our father came and told me that the war had begun, and, with sudden premonition and a feeling of sadness, I sensed that my world had changed. But more of that later. The other side of the orchard led to the chicken pen. There was a thatched summerhouse where my sister and I used to play.

Our father, Anthony Hanbury, dark, tall, and handsome, was a stockbroker, who made a daily commute to London, dressed in the city clothing of the time that included spats and a buttonhole with fresh violets. He was a passionate gardener—the vegetable garden was his domain—and he kept a small greenhouse where he raised scented cyclamens and Parma violets. Our mother, née Una Rawnsley, was blonde and beautiful and had grown up trained as a sculptor. She had spent some of her childhood on her parents' yacht and some of it in Italy. As a child, I remember thinking that our parents were surely the most wonderful people in the world, but in retrospect, during our early years, they were distant figures.

At the center of our world were our ponies. Jillian's Socks was a lovely bay Welsh pony, and my Cora was a New Forest pony that gave birth to a foal, Mayday, shortly after we acquired her. We were allowed to go off riding alone on the Commons that adjoined our property and in the nearby forest, Butterwood. We attended local horse shows and were taken foxhunting at an early age. Our mother went foxhunting regularly, at times three days a week, and on Saturdays both our parents hunted.

We had servants, sometimes varying in number. There was a pair of Irish maids, Kathleen and Gladys; two gardeners, one for the vegetable garden and one for the flower gardens; a groom, and once, briefly, even a butler, Sumpter. The two gardeners, Milhem and White, were remarkable

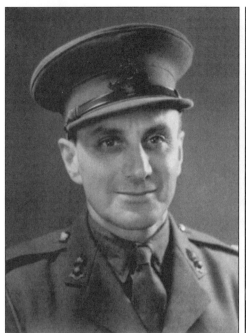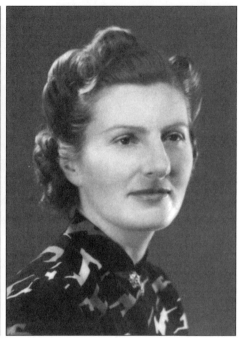

These are the photos of my parents that I was given to take to boarding school.

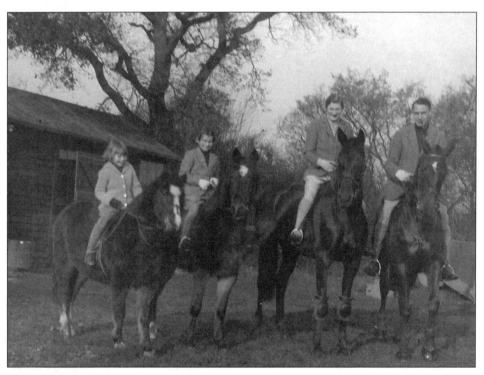

At Derbyfields in front of the stables. Jillian on Socks, me on Cora, my mother on Sutton Lass, and my father on Ripton.

in that White had fought in the Boer War and Milhem was one of the few people left in the county who knew how to thatch—I remember his rethatching the summerhouse one year. Pilbeam, who looked after the horses for a while, was married to a gypsy. Jillian and I were cared for by a series of governesses; first German, Annalise and Helme; and then, as tensions with Germany escalated, a French one, Aline Boulignat; and finally a wonderful Czech, Litzi Pisk, who taught us to paint. By the time I was eight, we were fluent in both French and German, and my sister and I spoke them interchangeably with English as we played together. We had no regular playmates. One family, friends of our parents with three children, would occasionally come down from London for a few days, and we attended birthday parties at the homes of two other children. But mostly, it was the ponies that were our companions. My sister was blonde, like our mother, beautiful and endearing, and was a favorite of all the governesses. I was unhappy, jealous, and, in retrospect, a difficult child.

When I was ten, we were sent to a day school that involved a short commute by train, and a year later I was off to a small and idyllic boarding school. My sister was home schooled, tutored by a wonderful Scotswoman who lived with her Air Force husband in a cottage at the foot of our pasture. My school, Brickwall, in Northiam, Surrey, was a small innovative school run by a dedicated woman whom we called Mog, short for Mogul. She had lived in India for many years. One of the first things she did for me was to teach me how to relax. As I lay on the edge of the swimming pool, she picked up my arms and legs and showed me how to let them go completely limp. Had I been able to continue at Brickwall, many of my later difficulties probably would have been resolved, and I would have gained confidence in myself. But this was not to be; by the time I turned sixteen I was to have attended ten different schools.

The day after my twelfth birthday, September 3, 1949, came too soon. We gathered in the sitting room to listen to the king's speech. George VI stuttered—as I learned later, dyslexia runs in the royal family— and we always held our breath hoping he would get through a speech without difficulty. I had been told that his speech therapist had him place three matches in front of himself; when he felt the stutter coming on, he was to rearrange them in a different order. Whether or not he was using this relaxation technique, I do not know, but he ended by speaking these words in a confident voice. I never forgot the quotation:

"And I said to the man who stood at the gate of the year,
'Where shall I find a lamp to lighten the darkness?'
And he replied, 'Put your hand into the hand of God and it shall
be for you brighter than a light and better than the known way.' "

The next day we went to the village hall, and I helped fill the sand-bags that were stacked around the windows. Our father was appointed air raid warden, and went about the village at night making sure that all the windows were totally blacked out. We were issued gas masks in little square brown cardboard boxes that we were supposed to keep with us at all times. Once, we went up to London and I saw the barrage balloons tethered above the city looking like great gray elephants. At school men from the local fire department came and showed us how to extinguish incendiary bombs; you had to use sand, never water. My school closed—it was too near the coast—and I was transferred to a large school, Benenden, where I was miserably homesick. A couple of months later, Benenden was evacuated to Newquay in Cornwall, where a hotel replaced the lovely old buildings and parkland. I became even more homesick. One morning I dreamed of Derbyfields and woke up crying. Throughout my school years it remained difficult for me to make friends—perhaps the result of our early isolation.

We spent part of the following year in the Lake District, in the north of England. My mother had inherited Dunnabeck, a slate cottage perched on the hillside above Rydal Water. The cottage was named for a nearby stream—the two Celtic roots mean "brown stream"—and many years later I chose this name for my summer camp. There Jillian and I spent some blissful months roaming the fern-covered fells, playing in the stream, riding our "stick horses"—substitutes for the ponies we missed—and bird watching down by the lake.

Our great-grandmother, Edith Rawnsley, lived in nearby Grasmere in her house, Allen Bank, and I admired her determination and strength from the beginning. She took in refugees from London—my sister remembers them screaming as the maid gave them what may have been their first bath. She offered shelter to a Jewish refugee couple, the Wieners, and found them a job caring for Dove Cottage, Wordsworth's home. She bicycled off to the village to meet the architect who was to install bathrooms in some cottages. She learned to cook—for after a while there were no servants—and to subsist on what food was available by creating delicious savory vegetable custards. I think she was my first real role model.

During this period our father had joined the artillery as a captain, but was soon to be invalided out because of a heart condition. He went back to the business world, where he prospered for a while. Conditions in England were getting worse. Even Churchill was convinced that England would be invaded. Our great aunt Ethel died and left our mother a sum of money—we never knew the exact amount—but she immediately

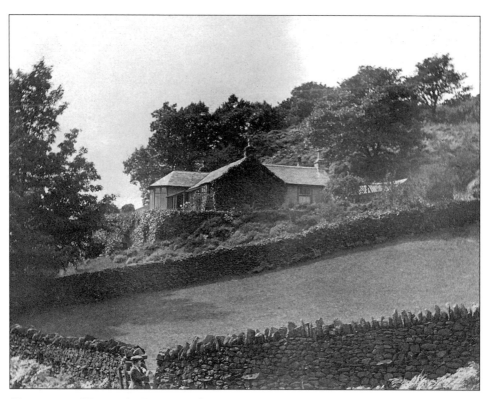

Two views of Dunnabeck, named for the stream that flowed nearby.

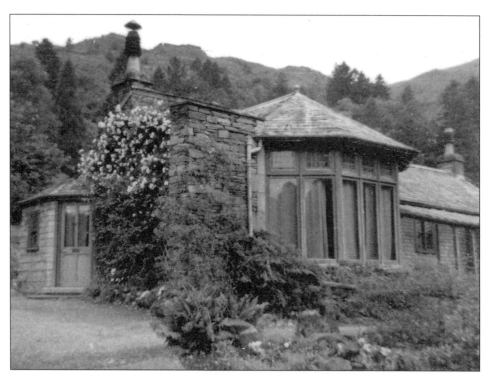

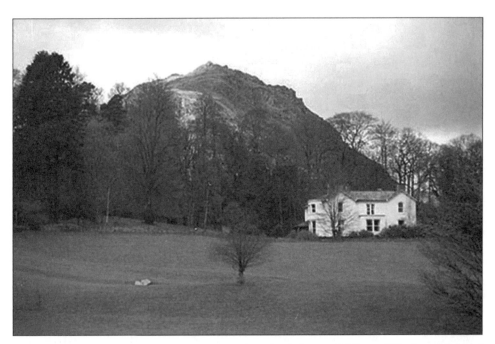

Allan Bank, in Grasmere, my great-grandmother's home. William Wordsworth lived there with family and friends from 1808 to 1810.

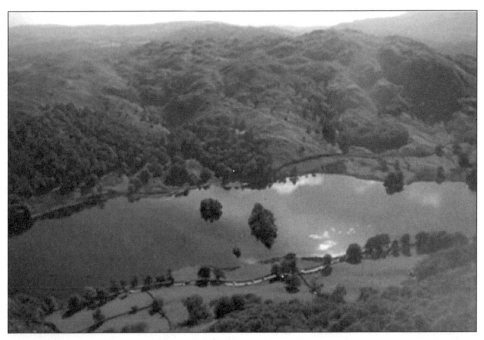

Rydal Water, which Dunnabeck looked down on. My sister and I were allowed to roam this lovely countryside by ourselves.

determined to take us out of the country to Bermuda for the duration of the war. In due course we embarked on what became a long voyage as we were zigzagging to avoid German U-boats. I saw my first iceberg, shining in the early morning light. We had to carry our life jackets with us at all times, and they were the heavy cork type.

We landed in Montreal where, for inexplicable reasons, I was left with a Canadian family while my sister and mother went on to Bermuda. The Boyds were a great family with a little three-year-old daughter, Nancy, whom I adored. They wanted to do something to help the war effort, and taking me on was to be their contribution. During my time in Canada they paid all my expenses. They soon arranged for me to have my tonsils out; I still remember the sore throat that lasted for days. I started in a day school in Montreal, where I had difficulty with all the schoolwork, even French, for my schooling had not included the conjugation of obscure verbs in the subjunctive mode. My grades were all D's, but unfamiliar as I was with the grading system, I did not understand what that meant. I was then transferred to Riverbend, a boarding school in Winnipeg, Ontario, where a group of students from Benenden School had been evacuated. I still remember the long train journey across Canada and the endless flatland followed by interminable pine forests. Winnipeg was cold—once forty degrees below zero—and the school was on the bank of a river, always cold and damp. Once more, I was homesick and friendless, worrying about our father in England, and missing both my parents and even my sister. At the end of the year, the school decided that they no longer wanted my presence. In answer to my mother's plea, they wrote back that after all, they had to "consider the other girls." I still do not know what I did to get myself expelled, but I do remember once leading a group of girls down the fire escape in the middle of the night.

And so I went to Bermuda to rejoin my mother and sister. My mother had settled into a glamorous life, enjoying the company of the Americans posted there, dancing on the terrace at the Coral Beach Club, swimming in the warm turquoise waters and working at Admiralty House. We lived in a series of wonderful white-roofed houses, moving, as I remember, at times because the water supply (Bermuda is entirely dependent on rainwater) ran out. My sister attended a day school in Hamilton, and I went off to a small boarding school, Somers College, at the far end of the island. As usual, I was rather quick to alienate my fellow students, but was rescued from misery and isolation by one of the teachers, Charles Violet, who taught me to sail and encouraged me in my life goal—to be the first woman to circumnavigate the world single-handed. Joshua Slocum was my idol. First I had a dinghy; then, with his encouragement, I acquired a Snipe. Painted red and named the *Phoenix*, she was the replacement for the horses and ponies that I still missed. The inland waters and coves of the sound provided plenty of safe sailing. I was exempted from sports—hard as I tried, I could never really master the field hockey about which my fellow students were passionate—and allowed to spend my afternoons sailing. On weekends I threw a duffel bag into the boat and sailed home across the sound. Our mother never seemed to worry about my safety, but on one occasion when I was becalmed and late in returning, she did phone the coast guard. I had started to paddle back, quite unfazed by the fading light. Sometimes on weekends we put on our homemade dirndl skirts and bicycled down to the U.S.O. in Hamilton. It was there that I met my first love, a young sailor off the French submarine, the *Surcouf*. Later, she was rammed accidentally by an allied ship and went down with all hands. I was heartbroken. For years I kept his letters and the little sketch he had made me of his ship.

Then I was off to another school. This time it was back to Canada, Toronto. My mother had taken a lot of trouble to make sure I would be suitably clad, and I remember a couple of outfits with dropped waists and matching hats, one plum and the other light green silk with little zebras on it, specially made for me. Alas, these alone were enough to set me off from my fellow students. I think we flew to New York—there were several other returning students—and then I took a train to Toronto. A taxi dropped me off at the school—no one had met me—and there I stood by the imposing doorway for a moment, thinking, "once again a lot of people who will not like me and with whom I can never make friends." And I was right. My English accent immediately set me apart. When the girls in the dormitory shrieked over letters they had received from their boy friends, which they were quick to share with the whole group, when they screamed every time Frank Sinatra came onto the radio, and when they wore makeup and jewelry, I was horrified. My only consolation was in studying. I was always weak in algebra, but very good at geometry, history, and languages—my mother arranged for me to substitute German for the physics and chemistry that were causing me difficulty. She came up to visit once, and we went to Niagara Falls. By this time she had left Bermuda— my sister had contracted yellow fever and needed better medical care— and settled in Washington, D.C. I was to visit her there briefly. Jillian was away at school, so that I had my mother all to myself.

It was very hot in those days before air-conditioning, and we slept on the roof. Early in the morning when we woke up, she taught me how to draw horses. I loved poetry, and she gave me a Louis Untermeyer anthology. On the flyleaf she inscribed a verse that reflected her abiding faith in my ability to do anything I wanted—go off horseback riding alone, roam the mountains in the Lake District, sail a boat, and certainly, if I wished, circumnavigate the world single-handed. I still have the book, and the verse:

One man with a dream, at pleasure,
Shall go forth and conquer a crown;
And three with a new song's measure
Can trample an empire down.

Somehow, even though the war was not over, it was decided that I would return to England for more challenging educational opportunities and live with my father in London before going off to college. I had looked forward to being with my father, but this was not to be. He had acquired a mistress, Claire, and our antagonism was mutual. Once I threw a teacup at her—cup, saucer, tea and all. I was moved into a boarding house and enrolled in a "crammers" for a program of intensive tutorials. Study became my passion. I often worked until three in the morning, and sometimes all night. I had wonderful tutors in French, German, history, and English, and they inspired me.

My very first night in England, there was an air raid alarm. Rather than take refuge in the basement, my father took me up onto the roof, and there we watched my first buzz bomb. It appeared as a luminous object making its way across the sky with an audible humming sound. It came down with a loud explosion. My father remarked, "That is in the City. I hope to God it's not near the office." But it was—almost a direct hit. There were no casualties—the night watchman had just stepped out for a cup of coffee. The next day we went there. I remember filing cabinets that had ended up in the next room and shards of glass embedded in oaken doors. Then came the V2's, guided rockets. If you heard the explosion, you were safe.

We celebrated the end of the war together, my father and I. Everyone was dancing in the streets; we really believed that along with the bluebirds over the white cliffs of Dover, there would be "love and peace forever after." Finally we joined the crowds outside Buckingham Palace and waited for the royal family to appear on the balcony. Shortly thereafter, my father and Claire, whom he had married, left for Rhodesia, where his brother, my Uncle Mike, had a large ranch and raised cattle and tobacco.

I enrolled in Bedford College, a branch of the University of London, much to the distress of my mother. I was only sixteen, and she felt I should have spent another year and reapplied to Oxford. I majored in German and, because of my fascination with medieval and renaissance Italy, minored in Italian.

My very first summer in England, I stayed with friends of my parents near Manchester and had a job as a Land Girl. The war was still on, and women were needed to replace the men. German P.O.W.'s, who were driven to the farm every day in a truck, added to the labor force. Most of them were very young and friendly; we often brought extra sandwiches to share with them. I was able to put my German to use by explaining what it was the farmer wanted done. The work was physically arduous. After a day of harvesting potatoes, I could barely move. We also arranged sheaves of oats into stooks that the wind would blow down overnight if it was not done right; that happened once, and Farmer Morton was furious with us. Even with long-sleeved shirts my arms were raw and itchy from the work.

Then I had a summer in France, helping an elderly couple in the Auvergne. I learned to love that primitive and rural country. I was sent on errands that often involved walks of several miles to fetch bread or meat. The bread came in great round wheels, on which it was customary to make the sign of the cross before making the first cut.

The first summer that tourists were allowed in Italy, I enrolled in the Universita per Stranieri in Perugia, and spent a very happy summer improving my Italian. I think this was the first time in my life that I found friends, people who liked me. On some weekends we took the train down to Lake Trasimeno, dangling our feet out of the sides of the cattle cars that were the only available transportation. In the evening we strolled along the Corso Vannuci and danced at the Bosco del Usignolo. We took a plane to Rome, where we stayed in a monastery on St. Peter's Square and could hear the fountains from our bedrooms. We wandered around the Forum, and we went on down to Naples and Capri.

In England, another summer, a group of us rented a boat and sailed on the Norfolk Broads. I bought a fourteen-footer, joined the Royal Corinthian Yacht Club and raced on the Thames. All alone, I enrolled in the Sir John Cass School of Navigation and learned both celestial and coastal navigation. I was the only woman in the school, but the Scottish captain who headed it said I could be there provided I promised not to do what the only other woman ever enrolled had done: she had worn so much steel in her corsets that during the course in coastal navigation the compasses had gone haywire. My plan of being the first woman to circle the globe single-handed was still very much in place.

Life in England was difficult, and food was more of a problem after the war as the supplies of Spam (ubiquitous meat of wartime) disappeared. We learned to improve powdered eggs by adding a little mustard.

I assuaged my teen-age hunger with crumpets and bread and bacon drippings. In addition to the usual teen-age acne, I started to develop boils—on my legs, my breasts, and finally on my face—at which point I became sufficiently alarmed to seek medical help.

I graduated with an Upper Second (an Honors degree)—not bad considering the difficulties with which I was coping: loneliness and ill health, and the fact that, because of returning war veterans, the work had to be completed in three instead of the usual four years.

Almost immediately, I sailed for Cape Town and then traveled by train up to Rhodesia. Life with my father and Claire continued to be tense, but I found a soul mate in my uncle, Mike. As a young man, Mike had flunked out of Osborne, the British naval academy, and after a brief foray to Canada, ended up in the early 1930's in Rhodesia. Over the winter holidays—the seasons there are reversed—he hired me to tutor my two cousins, Yvonne and Ashley. Although I did not know it at the time, both children were severely dyslexic, as was their father. I enjoyed working with them, but did not really know what I was doing. Neither of them ever graduated from high school, although they both went on to lead successful lives.

The farm, named Kildonan, was a glorious spread of seven thousand acres on which my uncle raised a thousand head of cattle and grew tobacco. It was something of a model operation, often visited by dignitaries from abroad. And he had lovely horses. Mike's wife, Elaine, was a wonderfully warm person whom I came to adore. I fell in love with Africa—the flat, big sky country, the night noises, and the distant drumbeats. Now it is no longer Southern Rhodesia, but Zimbabwe, and the capital Salisbury is Harare. But about a year ago I looked at a detailed map and, much to my amazement, found a place marked Kildonan. Many years later, when it came time to name the school that Kurt Goldman and I were to found, I named it for the farm that belonged to my beloved dyslexic uncle Mike.

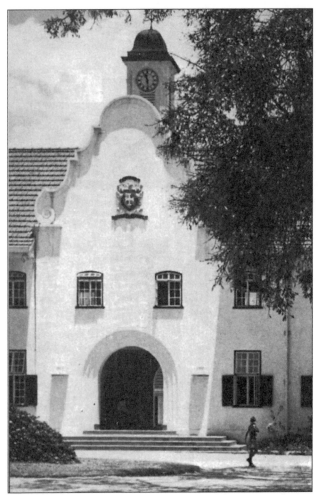

Left:
Ruzawi School was built in the lovely Cape Dutch style. I was there for only a year, but the experience changed my life.

Below:
Parrot Kopje. There were many of these in that region, and students were permitted to clamber all over them and to take dangerous leaps—a freedom no student would be permitted in our cautious society!

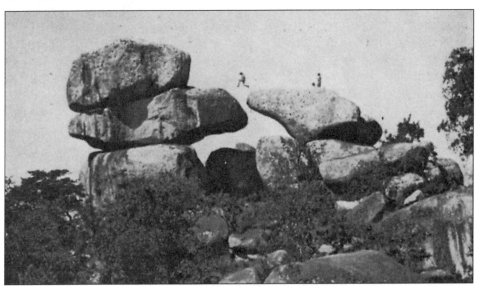

~ 2 ~

I Find My Vocation

Still I had no plans for what to do next in my life—a degree, even an Honors degree, in German and Italian is not preparation for any kind of career. My father had managed to secure me a promise of a job in charge of the rental department of a real estate agency. Then, the first miracle happened.

My aunt was shopping in downtown Salisbury when she ran into the wife of the assistant head of the Ruzawi School in Marandellas. She said, "We are getting desperate. School starts next week and we have no one to take the First Form." "Well," replied my aunt, "there is my niece…" Two days later I went there for an interview. The school was a beautiful campus of white Cape Dutch style buildings, with green lawns and playing fields set in rolling hills covered with msasa trees and dotted with piles of rock boulders called kopjes. When I got back, I remember thinking, "Please God, let me get this job and I will never ask for anything else for a very long time." Finally the phone—it was a party line—on the farm rang, and I was hired.

Ruzawi, founded in 1928 by Robert Grinham and Maurice Carver, was modeled after English preparatory schools. My charges were twelve small boys—they were supposed to have had their seventh birthday, but one of them was only six. They had been entered in the school at birth, or even sooner, at conception. They were known as the Kippers—a cross between Kids and Nippers—and came to board at school from all over the countryside. My classroom was away from the main complex and consisted of two large rooms, one of which we used for art and other projects. I taught everything, ranging from math and reading to history, geography and religion. I taught music—the only use I ever made of my many years of piano lessons—and in the early mornings before breakfast I led them in calisthenics and games of Simon Says, What is the Time Mr. Wolf, and Grandmother's Footsteps. I do not think I was very good as a teacher—I had neither experience nor training. But I was passionately in love with my job. The boys loved me, and the faculty liked me. It was a wonderful year. I was entranced by my young charges, with their fresh outlook on life and the unexpectedness of some of their responses. Once, a little boy spilled paint water on the floor, and when I asked him to mop it up, he refused, saying, "That is native's work." Then in a math lesson, I found one of them drawing a lion in his book. When I reprimanded him, he replied, "But, Miss Hanbury, it says to draw a lion three inches long." The boys were of course called by their last names, many of which I still remember. There was Frere who, when frustrated, would turn blue in the face and throw himself on the floor in a classic tantrum. I was reminded of my own childhood tantrums, when, as I later remarked, I could actually *see red*. Herbert, a very bright little boy, had especially lovely cursive handwriting—I kept samples for many years. There was Smith, who began the year as a non-reader, and then began reading *Dr. Doolittle* fluently. Fforde, still a six-year-old, but obviously brilliant, although his handwriting was messy. Cooksey, who had some health problems. Scott, who was, I now know, severely dyslexic. And Pyman who, about two years after I left, died suddenly of polio. We were expected to give them numerical marks for everything they did, and the totals and class rankings for the entire school were read out at the end of every term. For some reason Thurman had a low mark in religion, and his father, a minister, protested. I could offer no explanation. The school was modeled on English schools, and students were studying French by the second form and Latin shortly thereafter. While it was certainly strict—errant pupils were still caned by the headmaster—the older students were given a lot of both freedom and responsibility (never for other students, but for real tasks). They were allowed to roam the countryside and climb the kopjes, even leaping from rock to rock high in the air. They were Scouts and carried sheath knives, and they were trusted. I always remembered this way of dealing with teenagers, and, rightly or wrongly, always keep this model in the back of my mind.

At the end of the year, I was told that the school wanted me to stay on, but that they felt I should first spend a year taking a Froebel course at a school in South Africa—Natal, if I remember correctly. It was expensive, and I had no money. My father had lost most of his, swindled in a business deal by a partner whom he trusted—he never was a good judge of character. My mother was working to put my sister through college. While I was on the farm wondering what on earth to do, an English friend of my mother's offered to pay my fare to the States. My mother got me a promise of a job at The Potomac School on the strength of a photograph of me that she showed Carol Preston, the head. I had to go down to

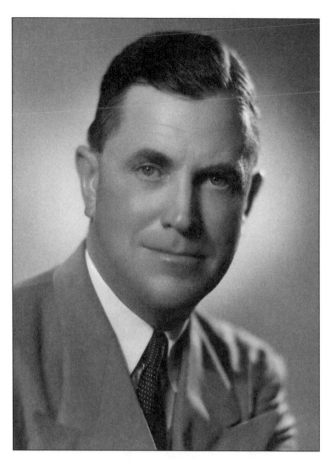

My beloved Uncle Mike, for whose farm Kildonan School is named. Had it not been for him and his wife Elaine, I might never have found my life's work.

Durban to get a visa, where I was asked to raise my right hand and swear that I had never committed any crime involving moral turpitude, had never been a member of the Communist Party, and was not a prostitute. I think I disconcerted the young foreign-service officer by giggling at this point.

The boat crossing lasted three weeks. It was a small cargo ship that carried only about a dozen passengers. Learning of my interest in navigation, the captain permitted me to participate. I was given a sextant and allowed to plot our position, and even to mark it on the chart, provided I initialed it. We shot four times a day: morning and evening stars, noon, and three o'clock sights. The stars were the most fun. They even sent a sailor to wake me for morning stars. In the evening you knew which planet you wanted to sight on, its elevation, and roughly where it would show up. You had to catch it quickly as you still needed to be able to see the horizon, so that you could bring the reflected image down and record the angle. You would then punch the stopwatch and walk with it in hand to the ship's chronometer. In making your calculation, you would subtract the stopwatch time from that of the chronometer. For morning stars, you would somewhat reverse the process by fixing on the planet and waiting until the horizon became visible. By the end of the trip, I was within three miles of our position. Navigation always seemed a miracle. But now, of course, it is all done by radio waves, and sextants are antiques.

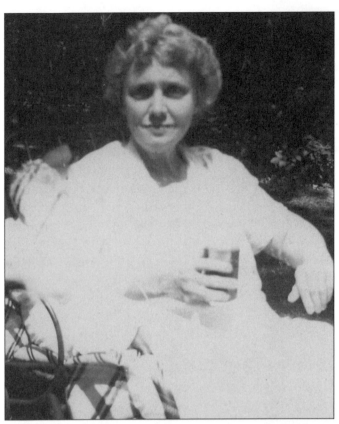

My mentor, Helene Durbrow, in 1939 at the beginning of her teaching career and, at a later date, with her grandson Mark.

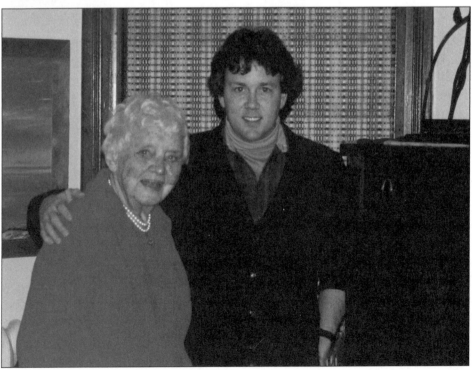

~ 3 ~

🌿 *Apprenticeship* 🌿

We landed in New York. I arrived in Washington, D.C. in the spring. The job that my mother had been promised for me did not materialize, as the school's new expanded quarters in McLean, Virginia, had not been finished. I applied to several schools and finally secured a summer job at Beauvoir, the elementary school from which the boys went on to St. Albans and the girls to National Cathedral School. I was the assistant in the kindergarten program. Right away I learned new, and I thought some of them silly, ways of handling children. For instance, you were not supposed to say, "Don't throw the blocks (or the clay)," but "Blocks are for building, " or "Would you like to make something with the clay?" When a child made a picture, you were not to ask what it was supposed to be, but rather to say, "Tell me about your picture." In Rhodesia I had read myths and legends that enthralled my young charges; here, they were supposed to read tales of neighborhood helpers— the policeman, the milkman, and the mailman—all of which I thought were unbelievably boring. The Washington summer heat was unbearable. When we could not sleep at night, we went to the movies, first checking to see which ones were air-conditioned. After the summer program ended, I was hired to stay on for the school year. I was there long enough to have to learn the routines of putting snow pants, jackets, and overshoes on our small charges. A dragon lady, Mrs. Taylor, ruled the school, and woe betide any faculty member who came into a meeting late. The only place where faculty could gather was in what we called the "gold fish bowl," a glass-enclosed space just outside her office. Then came another fortunate event.

One fine morning Robert Lyle, the head of Sidwell Friends School, and Frank Barger, the head of the Middle School, came to talk to Mrs. Taylor. They explained that they had a class of fifth graders that already had two teachers and was rapidly getting out of control. They wanted Mrs. Taylor to release me from my contract with her so that I could come immediately to take over that class. I am not sure why, although in hiring teachers I have noticed that British teachers often do have a knack for discipline.

I loved my class of twenty-eight boys and girls. They took to me immediately and named me "Miss Jolly Well Hanbury" because of my habit of saying, "You had jolly well better pay attention/do your home-work/sit up properly/etc." I stayed at Sidwell Friends for five years.

To my delight, the school was given a set of portable typewriters. All a teacher had to do was march the class up to the closet and collect them. I took greater advantage of these typewriters than did any other teacher. My students mastered the skill quickly, and began to turn out volumes of work. At one point I was even sufficiently skeptical to phone a parent and ask whether her daughter had really done this work all by herself. To my great relief, she indeed had. I learned that keyboarding facilitates written expression, even on a manual typewriter.

But there was another aspect to the school that quickly attracted my attention. Robert Lyle and Frank Barger were interested in the problems of strephosymbolia—a Greek compound meaning "twisted symbol" that Dr. Samuel Orton had coined to describe the reversal tendencies that often characterize the dyslexic. He had hired a Vermonter, Helaine Durbrow, to administer the program. Miss Anna Gillingham made four visits a year to supervise what was called the Language Training Program. Students enrolled in it spent as much time as was needed in tutorials in a separate building. At first they joined their classes only for sports, music, art, and perhaps math. As their skills improved, they were able to partici-pate in science, English, and social studies. Once a week Helaine Durbrow met with the teachers of each grade—there were two classes at each level of the middle school, which included grades five through eight. Miss Gillingham's visits were always intimidating. I remember her as a heroic figure, always dressed in black, and given to epigrammatic pronounce-ments such as, "What the teacher hasn't taught, the child doesn't know" and, in response to questions about pacing, "Go as fast as you can and as slow as you must." Once she was invited to speak to a group of teachers at a Baltimore private school. At the end of her lecture she asked for ques-tions. When one teacher timidly raised a hand and posed a question, Miss Gillingham harrumphed and said, "Young lady, if you had been paying attention to what I said, you would not need to ask that question." Needless to say, there were no further questions. Helaine Durbrow was terrified of her.

At the end of the school year, Helaine offered me a job at Camp Mansfield, the summer program she ran for dyslexic children. Located on a farm near Essex Junction, Vermont, it was a lovely piece of land—open fields, birch woods, and hills the glaciers had sculpted. A mountain stream ran through it, and to one side was a small ski area with a rope tow. The nearby warming hut was the boys' summer dorm. My teaching room was a corncrib. I spent the mornings in tutoring and the afternoons in teaching riding. Her daughter-in-law, Betsy Westervelt, acted as camp nurse and was there with her two young boys, Mark and Van. Her son, Bill Durbrow, and his wife Emmy were also there, Bill as Camp Director. Bill was severely dyslexic, and when he hadn't learned to read, his mother had taken him to Dr. Orton. She had no money, but Dr. Orton, with characteristic generosity, taught her how to teach him, and every month she went back to learn what to do next. This is never an ideal situation—there are many strictures against a parent's becoming the child's tutor, but nevertheless, it is sometimes the best workable plan, and I have often since mentored mothers in that task. Despite his success in adult life, Bill, as do many dyslexics, bore the scars of his early learning failures. He was quick-tempered when crossed, and everybody knew better than to beat him at a game of cards.

I was to spend three happy summers at Mansfield. During my last year at Sidwell, I worked in the Language Training Department with Jane McClelland and Mary Helen Robinson. The latter went on to found a school for young dyslexic children in Seattle—The Hamlin Robinson School.

My professional life was a happy one, but my social life was non-existent. My beautiful and socially adept sister and mother had numerous friends and glamorous parties and dates, and, despite their efforts to include me, I had none. It was the era of the cocktail party—an ambiance in which, to this day, I am ill at ease. Consequently, I took refuge in what I knew I was good at. I enrolled in a master's program at George Washington University. To my fury, the Dean pointed out that I had never had a science course at the college level and that that would be a requirement. When I protested, he suggested that I was lucky not to have to meet other undergraduate requirements, such as athletics, and concluded with the comment that over-specialization was one of the causes of war. Given a choice between zoology and botany, I selected the latter. When I entered the class, I demanded to know what was the lowest grade that would enable me to pass the course. But to my surprise, I loved it. I had never looked at cells through a microscope before and found I was good at drawing what I saw. For years I kept my chart of the life cycle of ferns. The degree offered by the German department headed by Dr. Sehrt was not the literature that had been my undergraduate interest, but comparative Germanic philology. Having studied Old High German, Middle

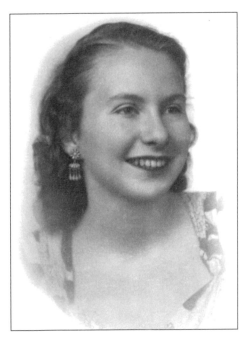

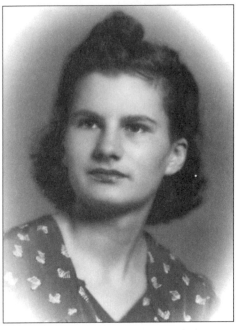

My beautiful sister. No wonder I was jealous of her!

The picture my mother took to Potomac School that got me a promise of a teaching job. At the time I was still in Rhodesia.

High German, and Gothic as part of my undergraduate program, I was exempted from some of the courses. Sanskrit, a two-semester course taught by Dr. Sehrt himself, was one I found especially challenging. This was a small class—there were probably five of us. It was in this course that I met James King. Jim had grown up in the depression years in Uniontown, Pa., had joined the army where he served in Germany, and had entered college under the veterans' program. I was attracted to his brilliant mind, impeccable scholarship, and wonderful sense of humor, and half a century later I can still appreciate these qualities. He loved me, I reciprocated, and in the fall of 1953 we were married in the National Cathedral.

Both of us had teaching jobs: I was still at Sidwell and he got a job at St. Albans. After finishing my day at Sidwell I often rode the streetcar down to the Library of Congress, where I worked on my M.A. thesis until the library closed, and then caught the last streetcar home. Our two children, Christopher and Sheila, were born twenty months apart, and I stopped teaching to look after them, although I continued to do some tutoring in the afternoons, especially while they napped. Unfortunately, our marriage did not last, and I finally left Jim one autumn. I still feel guilty about having done so, but also realize that our worlds were too far apart ever to mesh. We remain friends and talk on the phone about once a month. Our daughter Sheila went on to become a teacher and a poet and to have two children. She died of cancer in 2000, devastating all of us, but especially her two children, then aged twelve and sixteen. Christopher, our son, eventually moved to Albuquerque, where he married and embarked on a successful career in social work.

Once the children were a little older, I needed to find employment. A friend of mine had been offered the job of heading the remedial reading at The Potomac School. She did not take it, but suggested my name. To my delight Carol Preston hired me and offered me their top salary of four thousand dollars a year; moreover, Christopher could attend the newly established pre-kindergarten program, as could Sheila as soon as she was old enough—both of them on virtually full scholarship. I was to teach there until 1969. Both children had the best possible start in school. Potomac was a wonderful, creative, and vital place, full of activities and innovative programs. I am forever grateful for the generosity that made that education possible for them.

I enjoyed the school, but found less understanding of dyslexia than I would have liked. On one occasion, Dr. Lowry, the head psychiatrist at Children's Hospital, came to lecture to the faculty. He did all right, in my view, until he came to discuss the case of one severely dyslexic little girl who was a non-reader. He explained that her modern parents were in the habit of wandering around naked at their summer beach house, and that that sight had so shocked this child that she was afraid of looking at the words for fear of what she might see. I was longing to ask, but refrained, how he would account for her success in arithmetic. This was the era when psychological explanations were sought for dyslexia. According to one theory, the b's and d's so often reversed were sex symbols, and these children had unresolved sexuality. Later I ran across a discussion of a child who had difficulty, as some dyslexics do, with both math and reading. The explanation for that? Well, her mother was an editor and her father an accountant, and she was rejecting both of them. Dr. Orton had clearly established the link between brain structure and dyslexia, but his work was still little known outside medical circles. For many years I would continue to see children who had had years of psychotherapy but were still non-readers.

In those days Potomac School was more elitist than Sidwell, and enrolled the descendants of the Southern aristocracy and of Civil War icons, as well as the children of congressmen, senators, and judges. Carol Preston ruled the school with an autocratic hand, but her extraordinary intelligence and ability to understand children and, often, to find unusual

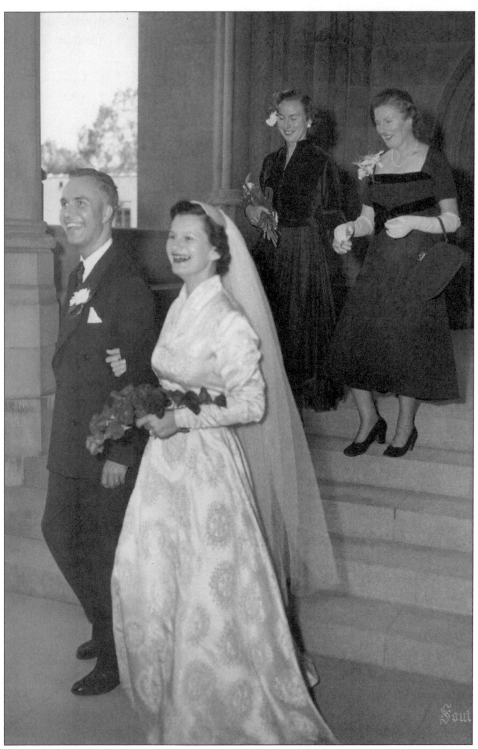

With Jim leaving National Cathedral in Washington, D.C., after our wedding. In the background, my mother and sister.

solutions to their problems provided me with an interesting role model. There are still aspects of her leadership style that I try to emulate.

My first work there was with younger children. I remember discovering that the fourth grade group was volatile, and a joke that would have amused my fifth graders at Sidwell set them off into helpless fits of giggles from which I could not retrieve their attention. Eventually, I moved to the upper school, where I had a room of my own. I had worked with older students in the summer, but this was my first experience in managing them in groups. I was good at it, and I loved the work. I taught the ninth graders speed-reading, then in vogue, using films that showed increasingly longer chunks of words at increasingly higher speeds. Soon all of them seemed to be reading at four to six hundred words a minute. There was also a speed-reading machine that lowered a bar over a page—the speed could be adjusted and the rate calculated by counting the number of words in a section of the page. This was the era of Evelyn Woods speed-reading courses, still in existence today. The theory was based on training of pilots during World War II. Instant recognition of aircraft, friendly or enemy, was crucial. An image of a plane would be flashed on a screen. At first the pilots would say they had seen nothing, but with practice their performance improved. I became one of the two eighth grade homeroom teachers and taught English. I also taught Latin to a group of seventh graders. But the most fun I had was with my ninth graders, in a class I devised in critical reading. Among other things, I taught them how to detect fallacies of all sorts—circular reasoning, argumentum ad hominem, flawed syllogisms, and so forth. As a final project, I had them find examples of each type in advertising and in things they heard people say. I like to think that some of them still retain the critical outlook that I tried to instill.

Potomac was good at giving dyslexic students the necessary accommodations, such as exemption from French and Latin, and in providing support services—me, and if necessary other tutors. By the time they reached the upper school, most of the dyslexic students could read, but continued to have great difficulty with written work. Tom Sayre, whose father and grandfather were dyslexic, had attended Beauvoir, where a friend of mine had taught him to read, but because of his dyslexia he was not eligible to enter St. Albans, despite the fact that his father was Dean of the Cathedral. I spent four years teaching him to write.

At the beginning of one summer Tom came to help me open the summer program. Within half an hour, he had produced two classic examples of the kind of speech error so very characteristic of the dyslexic: "What this place needs is a washerdisher," and "You should put a band-aid on that to keep the affection out." Tom went on to a successful career in outdoor sculpture—you can check out his website at thomassayre.com. About that time I was tutoring Peter Wright, who was later to become a renowned lawyer advocating for children with learning disabilities. As a child he drove his parents crazy by saying every single time he came into the TV room, "What's about that?" and one summer, he was told he had a new dentist, whose name was Dr. Armstrong, and forever Peter called him Dr. Strongarm. These little slips and spoonerisms are funny, but often signal underlying dyslexia. Later, at Kildonan, young students would ask me if I planned to "expect" their rooms. They always called the riding ring the "rink." Once, Charlie Kilgore, an excellent and daring skier, wrote an essay in which he described "power snow." He was highly incensed when I suggested that what he meant was "powder" snow. I began to understand how not knowing the printed word led to many such errors. In her old age, my mother's sight deteriorated—in her last years she was legally blind. We often traveled together, and she repeatedly mis-pronounced the names of places until I spelled them for her. Young Billy Durbrow, whose father had taught him the name for the breed of cow common in Vermont, was in the car with his father when he exclaimed, "Look Daddy, there's a steenhol!" Roger Saunders, a Baltimore psychologist, tells of a college student who opened a letter from the Dean telling her that she was receiving a "disgusting scholar award," and it took her a moment to realize her misreading. Not just parts of words, but entire words can be transposed. A student once called me to say, "You'll never guess what I said to my friends when we went to the theatre last night. 'Let's go after stage backwards.' They thought I was crazy, but I knew you would understand." These subtle speech errors often persist into adulthood. My hairdresser is energetic and artistic. When she first talked about feeling "flustrated," I put it down to lack of literacy, but then she continued to make little slips. My favorite—she is a staunch Catholic—was when returning from a cruise, she told her friends that the best part of the trip had been the visits to the "uninhibited" islands. She has two wonderful children, whom I watched grow up over a period of twenty years, and, sure enough, both of them are involved in the arts—one of the strengths of the dyslexic. Her daughter is already a gifted photographer, but a weak speller. Recently a parent, an engineer in his forties, told me he had driven north on the "Tectonic" Parkway.

Most dyslexics have a terrible time remembering names. Even with older students, we can read an entire book aloud together and be halfway through before they can correctly read the name of the protagonist. Dyslexia is a problem with language input as well as output. Often I find, especially in public schools, that the child is given tapes as an important accommodation. As anyone who has tried to learn a foreign language from listening to tapes can tell, auditory input alone is not enough, and for the dyslexic, this is especially so. While some of them do seem to have excellent vocabularies, many do not. It took us a while to figure out what was happening at mealtimes with one particular student. He never asked for food to be passed to him. He was afraid that if, for instance, he were to ask for broccoli, someone would laugh, and say, "You mean the spinach!" Better to go hungry than to be thought stupid. When I taught at Sidwell, I had made my fifth graders learn reams of poetry. When I started to teach our dyslexic students literature, I thought anybody who tried could surely memorize "Stopping by Woods on a Snowy Evening." I soon discovered my mistake.

If there are these problems with English, their native spoken language, one can readily imagine the challenge a foreign language can pose. Dyslexic students can fail French—harder than Spanish or German—as often as anyone is willing to let them continue to try. Canadian students could almost never gain exemption from the French required for college entrance. In this country, interestingly enough, Harvard was the first university to recognize that there were bright and valuable minds that could never master the foreign language requirement and had to be exempted from it. But even today, many independent schools insist that a child at least attempt the language. So, at times a young student is put into a Spanish class, for example, where the teacher is very good at teaching the sounds of the vowels, only one of which has any resemblance to the English sounds, thereby further complicating the job of the tutor. Again, I hear, "What harm can it do for him/her to at least give it a try?" To which my response has always been, "Hasn't this child had enough failure that you shouldn't have to ask, 'what harm is there in yet another failure?'"

Some dyslexic students do indeed master a foreign language. Perhaps later in life they join the Peace Corps: highly motivated, mature, and in a language immersion program, they do manage. My dyslexic cousin Ashley, when in high school at Michaelhouse in South Africa, asked to be allowed to substitute Zulu for the required French and Latin. He was taught by the caretaker and became completely fluent. I listened to him giving orders, conversing, and even joking with his farm hands in this complicated language, complete with its clicked sounds—his speech indistinguishable from that of a native speaker. So I have been told, for while I have heard him speak Zulu, I know only a few words of the language. At Baltimore Friends School, one teacher had success in teaching Spanish by using the sort of multi-sensory and structured approach that we use in teaching our dyslexic students English.

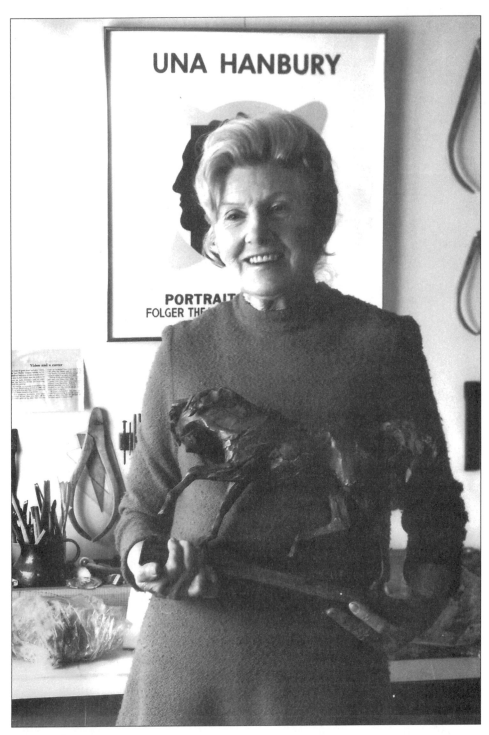

My mother, a sculptor, and supporter of all my aspirations, discovered the site that would become Dunnabeck.

~ 4 ~

❧ *Dunnabeck: the Beginning* ❧

One day in Washington, D.C. my mother ran into an old friend, Geoffrey Kitson. He was worried about his son Richie. The child had been born with a serious seizure problem—as a toddler he was having a seizure about every twenty minutes. Surgery to alleviate the problem had been performed in Montreal by Dr. Wilder Penfield, director of the Neurological Institute and a pioneer who specialized in brain surgery and in locating areas of specialization in the brain. Wilder Penfield was a remarkable surgeon, and a wonderful person. Molly Masland told me that once over dinner she had asked him what he thought was the single most important thing for him to do as Director; he replied that it was to "be generous" to those with whom he worked—and he did not mean money. The surgery had alleviated the seizures, but left Richie with a useless right hand and an awkward gait. But he was a bright little boy, and his failure to learn to read at all had been devastating to his parents. With the chutzpah of youth, I promised that if the family would pay my fare to Bermuda, I would come down and teach the boy to read during the upcoming Christmas holidays. And, in retrospect, to my great surprise, I succeeded. I worked with him for half-hour periods thrice a day, following the early Gillingham sequence, and by the end of my stay he was reading and writing—in nice left-handed cursive—a large number of three-letter words. The following summer, together with his nurse, Divey, he was enrolled in Camp Mansfield, the Vermont camp Helene Durbrow had established.

The very first summer program I ran was not actually in this country. In partnership with the Kitsons we operated Camp Messina in Bermuda, in buildings that had been part of the Dockyard. Half the students came with us by plane from this country and half were Bermudian. The instructional staff was American, and the counselors Bermudian. My husband Jim came along to help with the administration, as did my first-born son, Christopher, then just a year old. The swimming—we had our own dock—and sailing activities were wonderful.

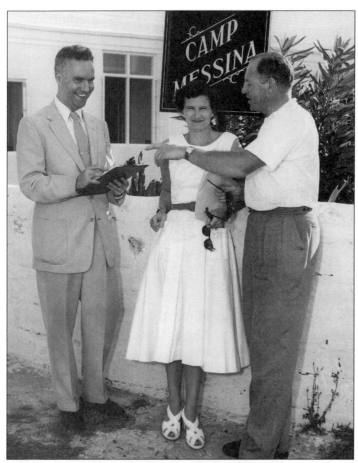

Left:
With Jim and
Geoffrey Kitson.

Below:
The group posing
for a picture.

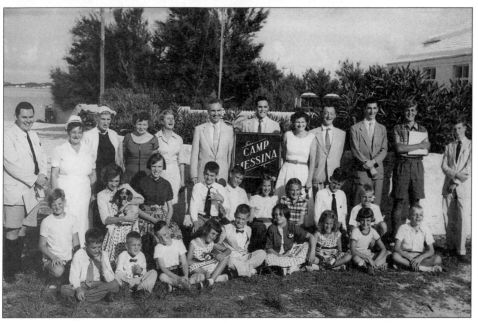

Aside from the children, we instructed an interesting adult. As a child, he had been forced to switch to his right hand, and now, whenever he had to speak on the phone and make notes, as his job required him to do, he developed a terrible stutter. It had been suggested that if he could be taught to write with his left hand, the stutter would disappear. We successfully retrained him, and, indeed, the stutter vanished.

I have two rather dramatic memories of the summer. A young counselor, despite our warnings never to do so, dove off the dock, deceived as to the depth by the clarity of the water, and came up with his face bleeding from coral scrapes. And, a little girl, Helen Flather, sat down on a prickly pear bush. The long spines, thoroughly embedded in her behind, had to be removed by a doctor in town. I held her hand, and as I watched the process with her clinging to me and saying, "Mummy, Mummy..." the room swayed and the nurse in attendance hastily produced smelling salts. I did not know that merely watching a child in pain could have this effect, but the experience was to be repeated later in my life. We had a successful summer, but I am never good at collaborative efforts. Probably my uncooperative attitude was exacerbated by the fact that I was pregnant with my daughter Sheila, who would be born the following February. I wish I could say that the Kitsons and I parted on amicable terms, but it was not until several years later that we were able to resume our friendship. However, one very important event came of our aborted collaboration. Betty Kitson was so greatly impressed by the help Richie had received that she decided to devote the rest of her life to the teaching of dyslexic students in Bermuda. She got her master's degree in reading from Columbia, and with help from Angie Wilkins established the Reading Center, first in her home and then in downtown Hamilton. Hundreds of children are helped by the tutors trained there, both at the Center and at other schools on the island. She was so successful in raising scholarship funds that no child has ever been turned away. A truly remarkable lady.

I had inherited seven thousand dollars from a trust fund established by my father, and I knew exactly what to do with the money. I wanted more than anything to establish a summer program for dyslexic students. It would, of course, be modeled on Camp Mansfield, the program established by my mentor, Helaine Durbrow. I wanted to place it in a rural setting far from the distractions of town and away from the heat of Washington, D.C.

I was still in hospital, where I had given birth to my daughter Sheila (in those days a week was not considered excessive hospitalization for childbirth), when my mother went to look at a piece of property. At that time she was remodeling and building houses and had in her employ a housepainter named Harry. Harry was from Western Pennsylvania, and mentioned that he knew of a property that was for sale and just might be affordable. My mother and Harry went to investigate. She brought back some pictures of little snow-covered cabins, a barn, and a large building, the lodge. Even better, she had already negotiated the price.

The property was owned by the Kiwanis Club of Brownsville, and had been built before World War II as a camp for underprivileged children from the local coal-mining towns. During the war, it had fallen into disuse. Later, it briefly became a football camp, and the cabins still bore the signatures of football players—some of whom would later become famous. By the time I bought it, it had stood empty for years. The price my mother had settled was ten thousand dollars, half to be paid at settlement, and the balance at the rate of a thousand dollars a year. This left us two thousand dollars for much-needed repairs and remodeling.

I did not see the property until late spring. It was on top of Mount Summit in the heart of the Laurel Highlands. Our ten-and-a-half acres lay in a small valley between the hills, and had a stream running through it. You crossed a bridge, drove along the side of a field and followed the red dog (as coal slag was called) driveway up to a red-painted barn and a long white building, the lodge. Behind the lodge were eight cabins, arranged in two rows of four. Aside from the field and the path between the cabins, later named the Fairway, the area was overgrown with the lovely wild mountain laurel—actually a plant that is rhododendron. It flowers in early summer—huge pink blossoms that turn white as they fade. The real laurel, known in those parts as "calico bush," covered the more open hillsides. It grew tall. Later, when I rode my horse along the trail, that laurel towered over my head. Ferns grew everywhere, especially the Christmas fern whose leaves reflect the light so beautifully. In the spring, we were to find patches of yellow ladyslippers—as many as twenty blooms in a clump—and even the rare pink ladyslipper. Several kinds of trillium filled the woods, and yellow dog-tooth violets flourished in the damp ground near the bridge. There was mayapple everywhere and skunk cabbage in a swamp. There was at least one patch of Indian paintbrush. In late summer fringed gentians bloomed along the path above the pool. Botanists from the University of Pennsylvania came occasionally in search of rare ferns. Once, a group came seeking permission to dig for mandrake roots. Huge boulders, a legacy of the ice age, were scattered everywhere. But the real glory of the place was the stream. Its waters were always icy cold. It ran noisily over rocks and formed pools and little waterfalls. In the spring it was overhung with fragrant white and pink azaleas. Because it reminded

Right: One of the cabins, when my mother first saw the property in February of 1956.

Below, center: A camp group in 1956.

Bottom: View from the entrance. The lodge is on the right and the barn on the left. The eight cabins were ranged behind the lodge.

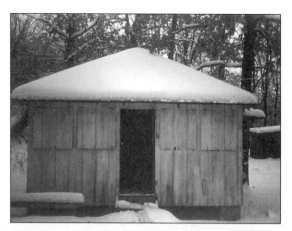

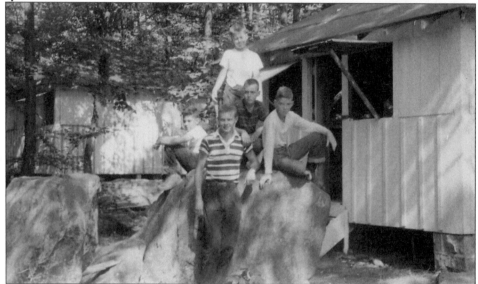

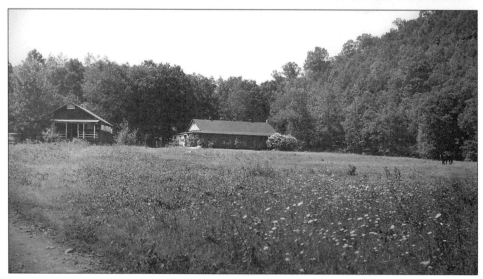

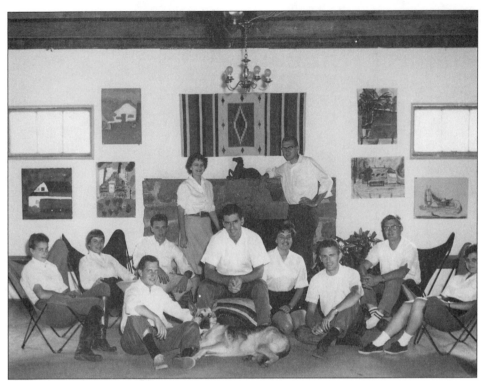

Above: Staff members posed around the lodge fireplace. On the left in riding britches is Ann Spiegelberg, now Ann Brown, and a valued faculty member at Kildonan. Shirley Kokesh is seated next to her. I am standing with Paul Biskup, head counselor. Below: The lodge porch was used for meals, and for study for the younger campers.

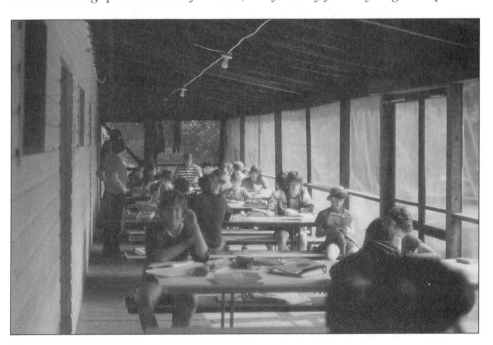

me of the stream in the English Lake District where I had played as a child, I named it and the camp Dunnabeck. The climate was rain forest—rain and mist all summer. The nights were always cool. I was to spend twenty-seven summers of my life in that environment, and occasionally, I still dream of it. But I have never been back.

There was much to be done to get ready for our first summer. Everything needed painting, especially the eight cabins. They all needed re-roofing. Some of the shutters that were nailed shut in the winter and propped open on poles in the summer had broken hinges. Everything needed re-screening. My mother undertook, and largely supervised, a huge project—the dry walling of the inside walls of the lodge. She taught me how to find the studs and how to do the nailing and taping. There was a hole in one corner of the lodge floor that we could not afford to have fixed for several years; we simply arranged a bunch of rhododendrons over it. At one end of the lodge was a large fireplace with a stone mantel and a chimney that went all the way up to the rafters. We hung a Mexican rug above the mantel, put a rug in front of the fireplace and arranged brightly colored butterfly chairs in front of it. In the middle we put a large oak table with a wonderful Indian-made basket that we always kept filled with branches of rhododendrons or bunches of wild flowers. The far end was the kitchen, separated from the larger room by a counter. Two doors to the back opened onto the Fairway, and a wide door facing the field led to a screened porch that ran the length of the building. This was our dining room, and we painted the tables and benches bright green.

Water came from a spring high on the hillside. Only the lodge had electricity, and water ran only to the kitchen and the shower house. The shower house was a concrete floor with corrugated metal sheets for the roof and walls. But it had a wonderful view of the stream that ran behind it. Beyond the cabins were the "brunos," as we named the outhouses.

We lived out of doors. We ate on the screened porch, slept in screened cabins and breathed the mountain air day and night. Some of us found it difficult to fall asleep in an enclosed space when we went back home at the end of the ten or twelve weeks. Often we awoke to early morning mists, watched the changing weather that governed our activities, and wandered off to bed by moon or starlight, carrying flashlights on pitch-dark nights.

Horses and riding were always an important part of the program. Having grown up riding and loving horses, I thought it was an important part of childhood, and that mastering the requisite skill would give these children a special sense of accomplishment. Every camper rode every day during the morning in the riding ring that we fenced in at the bottom of the field. The first summer we had a single pony, the following summer two horses, Midnight and Star. Finally, with the help of a generous parent, we built a stable. Then we added two small paddocks and had ten or twelve horses and ponies. We paid a few of our "seniors" to help care for the horses. This job involved getting up—sometimes by five in the morning—to get the horses fed, tacked up, and ready for the early morning trail rides. In the evening, on days when there was a late trail ride, the stable crew was ready to help cool off, untack, and water and feed the horses, sometimes by moonlight. We rode all over the countryside, even around the grounds of Fort Necessity, until the Park Service put a stop to that. The morning trail riders usually carried breakfast with them, and the evening riders always had a special picnic. Wonderful riding instructors, including my mother, Mary Stuart, Penny van Hoover, and Ann Spiegelberg, made sure that the horses were properly cared for and that everyone learned to ride English style.

The first summers we swam in a pool across the road from the camp. It had no filtering system, and we simply dumped chlorine in it. Then a parent, Bill Scarlett, lent us the money to build a pool of our own. We placed it on the hillside above the camp. An area of short grass surrounded it and a huge boulder, excavated as part of the process, was set on the side and became a favorite sunbathing spot. On the fence around the pool I grew purple and white clematis. Later we installed lights, and nighttime swimming became a favorite activity of both campers and staff. Skinny-dipping was popular, and we hung a flag to warn female staff away when the boys were swimming in the nude. Lit at night, the pool water was clear turquoise, and one could imagine oneself on an island resort. But the water was always cold, especially in the mornings, and one young camper from the Caribbean never understood how we could swim without wetsuits.

After a while commercial groups began offering raft trips down the Ohiopyle River. That section of the river was wild and rough, and no children under twelve were allowed to sign up. But for the rest of the campers the raft trip was the highlight of the summer. The rafters were equipped with life vests and helmets, and carefully instructed in safety procedures. The young guides were proficient, and one of them always followed in a kayak. While occasionally someone fell out of a raft, there were no injuries and no serious mishaps. At the end of the trip, the rafters piled into a bus and were driven back to the starting point. I went once myself, and found the experience rather terrifying.

The Youghiogheny Dam formed a wonderful clear lake, narrow but several miles long. We bought a boat and incorporated water skiing into

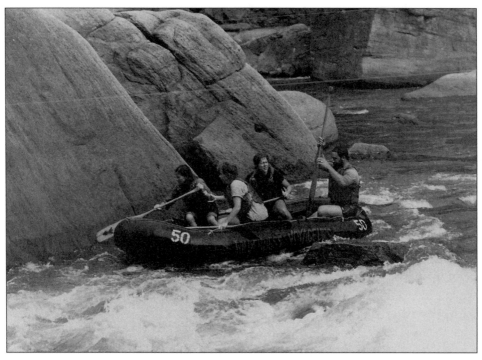

My one rafting venture—but notice I am the only one doing anything about the situation!

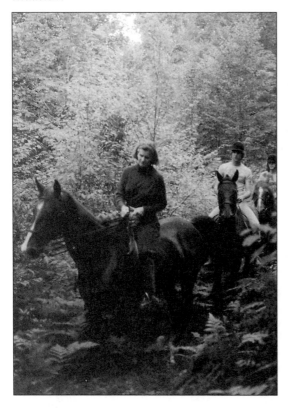

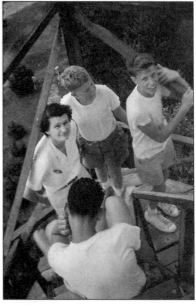

Leading an evening trail ride and another group to the top of a nearby firetower.

our program of weekend activities. Early in the morning we would set out—the dam was a forty-minute drive away— with the first group. Half of us would start skiing—the water was perfectly still at that time of day. The other half of that first group would be making breakfast at one of the campfire sites—always grilled steak and eggs. After breakfast, the rest of the group would ski. We had lunch at The Toll House, a short distance from the dock. Then the bus would come, bringing the afternoon skiers and picking up the morning ones. We skied all afternoon and always stopped by The Toll House for their homemade pie—rhubarb and strawberry was a favorite but they had several kinds—before returning to camp. Sometimes we took a few extra pies back. For many years I was the water-skiing instructor, but eventually we hired people who were better qualified.

As anybody who has run a school knows, while teachers and students are important, the cook is the kingpin one cannot do without. Perched as we were on top of Mount Summit, getting someone who would brave the early morning mists was always a challenge. Nevertheless, we had some great cooks. My mother did most of the cooking one summer. Anna Larkin, my stepsister still in college, managed amazingly well another summer. One remarkable summer we had a succession of six cooks. The first one quit before the campers arrived and, according to the amused health inspector, promptly reported us for feeding the cats and dogs from the same dishes we used for people. There followed a series of very nice competent ladies, public school cooks, who didn't mind helping out, but did not want to work in the summer. At last we hired a splendid cook, but she broke her leg on the second day. At that point I promoted the dishwasher to cook, and we got through the summer.

Finally, we found "Mom," as everybody called her. A tall motherly lady, she delighted in feeding the camp group. She had had no professional training, but had cooked for groups of hunters every fall and was certainly up to the job. Among my favorites was "halupki," a Polish dish of rolled cabbage leaves stuffed with meat—the campers probably liked her huge slabs of chocolate cake the best. In the middle of every morning she always made donuts for the Senior boys, who had to spend the entire morning in study. We enjoyed this treat, washed down with a couple of gallons of milk, out on the deck of my teaching cabin. We leaned over the railing and fed crumbs to the crayfish in the stream below.

It took us a while to find the sources for wholesale food. In the early years, I drove down the mountain to Uniontown to do the shopping in the afternoons. Eventually, we found how to arrange for most of it to be delivered. A huge freezer held much of the meat supply for the summer.

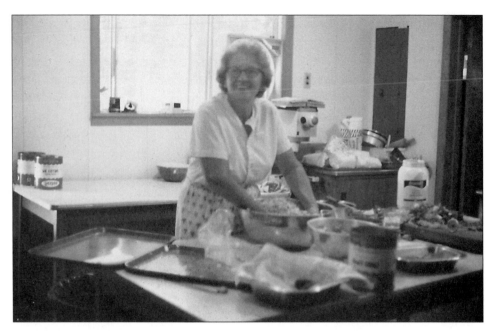

"Mom" in the kitchen.

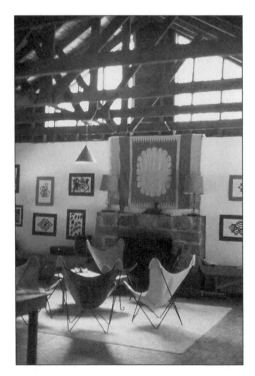

Lodge interior after we added windows.

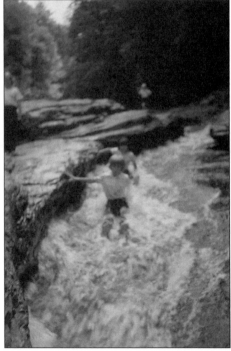

Ohiopyle slide, where generations of campers and staff wore out their blue jeans.

The first year we relied on an ice-box, until I found out that ice for the summer cost more than a refrigerator would have. Finally, we purchased an enormous refrigerator that came out of the Pentagon, where they were apparently doing some remodeling. Ken Brown, who had joined our staff as business manager, brought it back in his truck, and it served us well for many years. The first summer we relied on a wood stove. One of the counselors used to get it started before setting off down the mountain to pick up the cook.

Then there was Dalton and his wife Vi. Dalton served as our handyman from the beginning. He had been injured in a road-building accident when someone had set off the dynamite at the wrong time and sent him flying up in the air, and he was on welfare for the rest of his days. He mowed the field, built fences, painted and re-roofed, and kept an eye on the place in the winter. He and Vi had a large family of children, several of whom we got to know. I picked up his habit of calling a bag a "poke," a word I had only encountered before in the expression, "a pig in a poke." He delighted in bringing bad news with the preamble, "I knowed it. Just as soon as I seed it, I knowed it." Vi washed the dishes for many years and helped with the cooking. They lived a few hundred yards from camp in a relatively primitive little cabin. To Vi's great pride and joy, Dalton eventually built her a bathroom, complete with bathtub.

The camp never made money. I was no good at financial management, never planned a budget, and every year worried about being able to pay the last of the bills. Nevertheless, every year we improved what we had or added new buildings. We bought another fifty acres. When we first purchased the property, there were eleven buildings: the barn, the lodge, eight cabins, and the shower house. By the time we left twenty-seven years later in 1982, there were twenty-four buildings. The larger additions were my teaching cabin, the senior lodge, the infirmary, and the art barn. Smaller buildings included cabins for staff members, Senior cabins for our oldest campers on the far side of the creek, the stables, the tree house, and my sleeping cabin. Others were re-modeled. We added tutoring rooms built onto the lodge, put windows into the cabins, paneled them, and even added toilets to two of them.

A young architect designed my teaching cabin. It was cantilevered out over the stream. The sound of running water seemed to help concentration and masked the sound of my voice. I taught in one corner of the room and kept an eye on the ten or twelve students working at tables. Students who had finished their written work could move out onto the deck and read in beanbag or butterfly chairs. Years later I found out that the designers of medieval monasteries, whenever possible, placed the

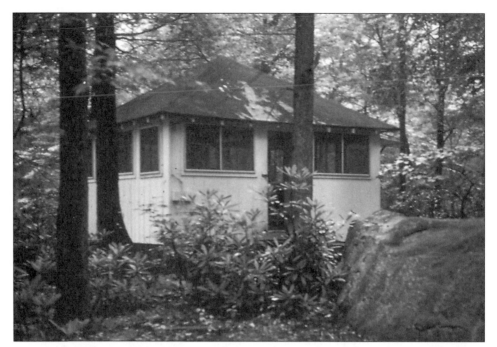

My first teaching cabin. Campers who got in trouble were sent to sit on "the Rock" until I had time to talk to them.

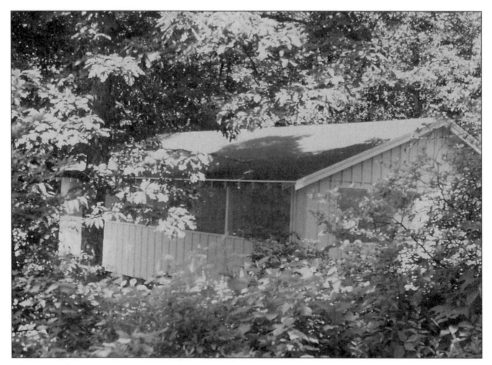

A view of my new teaching cabin.

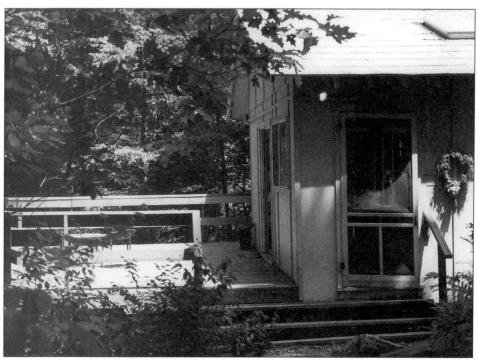

The deck to my new teaching cabin was cantilevered out over the stream.

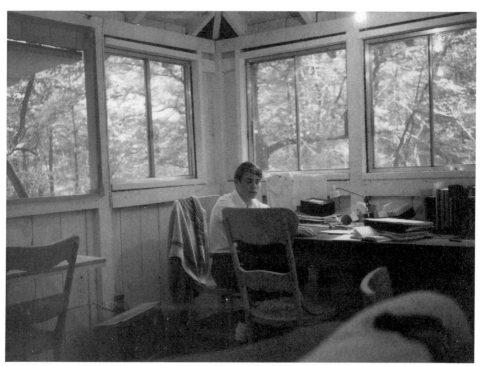

View from inside my teaching cabin with a student at work.

infirmary over running water, in the belief that invalids healed faster there. Perhaps it had something to do with the ozone generated by the running water. But, soothed by the sound of the stream, I could, and often did, tutor for eight hours a day without tiring. Early in the morning I would wend my way down the hillside, often walking into the dense mist, to meet my seven-o'clock student. Breakfast was at eight. I then tutored from nine to one, took a break until three (I am never at my best after lunch), and went back to work until six o'clock supper.

At first I slept in the little cabin—one of the eight—where I tutored. Then I bought an army tent and set it up on a platform on the hillside above the swimming pool. It leaked, and I spent several nights huddled under blankets hoping to fall asleep before the water soaked all the way through. The following summer, I had a little cabin built. The door opened onto a small deck, and a large picture window overlooked several tall tulip poplars beyond which lay the pool. At first, there was no electricity, but a hose supplied running water, and I added a little outhouse with a marvelous view—no need for a door.

Our senior boys and their counselor initially lived in a large cabin by the stream at the far end of the field. Later we built four little cabins on the far side of the creek, providing these sixteen- to eighteen-year olds with a measure of independence. At first they had to cross the stream to get there, but later we built a bridge, about which I will tell more later.

Art was always an important part of our program. Dyslexic students are often talented in the arts, and the activity made a good break from studying. Much sketching took place out of doors. When we built the art barn, we added a kiln and a couple of potters' wheels. Always we hired professional artists as instructors.

The infirmary with attached nurse's quarters was an ambitious project, built larger than necessary, because, until I saw the finished product, I did not realize how big it would be. For a number of years we had managed without a nurse—never a possibility these days. I relied on my experience raising my children and on my common sense. We were fortunate. In all the years, nothing really serious ever happened. But we had some close calls.

On one Saturday the camp was deserted except for seventeen-year-old Andy Faust, the son of one of our teachers, who stayed behind to look after a young boy who, for whatever reason, could not participate in the planned activities of the day. The child was stung by a bee. Andy checked the medical records, which included some allergies, but a statement to the effect that he was "not allergic to bee sting." The child complained that he felt dizzy, but then he was something of a malingerer. However, Andy looked at him closely, then put him in the car and drove the ten miles to Dr. Kamons. By the time they got there, the doctor commented, "Another twenty minutes and it might have been too late."

Knowing our situation, Dr. Kamons took the time and trouble to instruct me in some basic procedures that he felt might be important. He was careful to make sure that I understood how to diagnose appendicitis. One night, about two a.m., I was awakened by a counselor who reported that one of his charges had been throwing up and complaining of abdominal pain. Using the skills in which I had been coached, I decided that this was probably appendicitis, threw a raincoat over my pajamas, and headed down the mountain for the hospital, where we waited for a long time in the emergency room. The young doctor on duty was reassuring. "Whatever this is," he said, "it is certainly not appendicitis." Not entirely reassured, I explained that I was *in loco parentis*, was responsible for my camper, and asked him to do a blood count. "Lady," he replied, "we decide who gets blood counts." At seven o'clock, the house surgeon came in, took one look at the patient, and had the appendix out within half an hour. The director of the hospital could not have been more apologetic.

Another time a group of hikers came back with one young boy screaming in pain. Somehow and unaccountably, they had had a mud ball fight, and he had been hit in the eye. I laid him down on the ground and directed a stream from the hose into his eye until the last vestiges of the mud had been forced out—almost certainly a risky procedure, as I look back on it, but at the time I did not know what else to do. We were ten miles from the nearest doctor and an equal distance from the hospital.

Then there was the bridge disaster. We decided to build a bridge across the stream at a fairly wide point across from the senior boys' cabin. We were given four sections of steel I-beam. The plan was to lay planks over them lengthwise and then to place shorter planks at right angles to these. An "expert" assured us that the I-beams did not need to be riveted, but merely welded. Under the supervision of one of the counselors, the boys set to work with enthusiasm, devoting any free time they had to the project. Then, one day, the entire structure collapsed. Only by the grace of God was nobody under it at the time. We had the beams professionally riveted, started over, and the bridge lasted, and, for all I know, is still standing.

My children, Sheila and Christopher, loved Dunnabeck. Sheila was still a baby and Christopher, 20 months older, was still a toddler the first summer. I hired someone to look after them while I was teaching, and as they grew older, they participated in more and more of the camp activities. Christopher became an avid horseback rider. He especially enjoyed

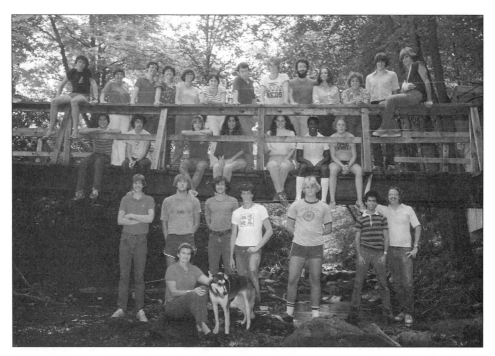

The bridge that collapsed during construction. Senior campers and staff posing. I am sitting on a rock, not under the bridge!

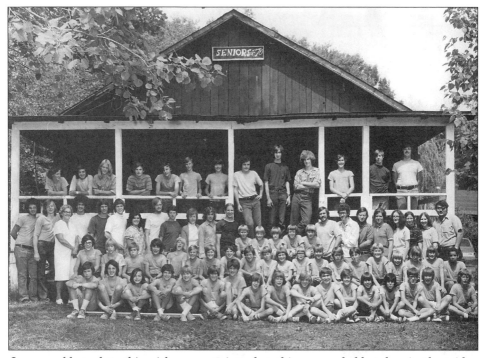

I am unable to date this with any certainty, but this was probably taken in the mid-seventies.

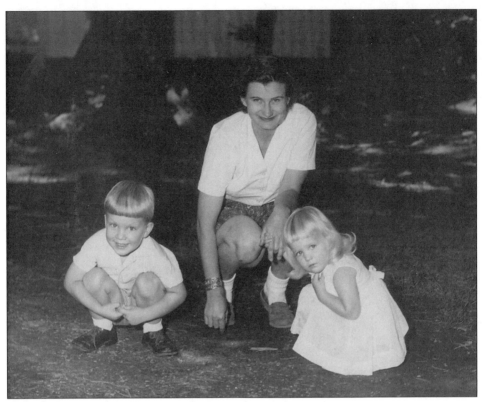

Above: The first summer at Dunnabeck with Sheila and Christopher. Below: My favorite steed, Fella, was a quarter horse that had been trained in barrel racing.

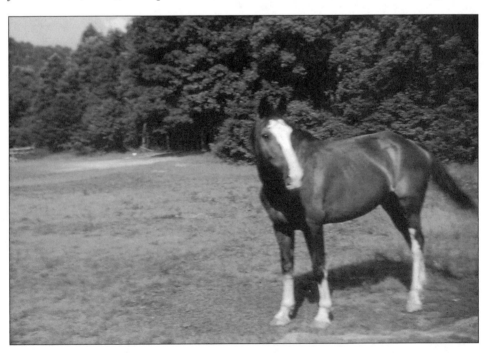

learning to jump under Penny's instruction. Sheila above all loved wandering in the woods, finding wildflowers, red efts (the baby newts), and a rock on which to sit and read. One summer I hired Carl Sandburg's granddaughter to look after her, and that may be when she first developed the love of poetry that became her lifelong avocation. As they grew up, they became a part of the camp staff. Both of them eventually tutored expertly. Christopher became first a counselor and then, his last year, head counselor, and began to develop the skills that eventually resulted in his career as a licensed social worker.

After camp, the whole family—my mother, my sister, her husband, and their two children—as well as one or two friends, came up for a couple of weekends of relaxation. We swam in the pool, rode the horses, and explored the woods, often going our separate ways during part of the day. I discovered that Richard, Jillian's husband, was an excellent rider, really the only person able to manage Fella, my beloved quarter horse. A magnificent steed, he was my pride and joy. He was black with a white stripe and four white legs. He had been trained in barrel racing before I got him, and at the slightest shift in position he would leap into a full gallop.

We opened the first summer with seven campers. This was not enough to make ends meet. While enrollment was always a concern, by the last summer we were enrolling nearly fifty. From the beginning we kept the younger campers on one schedule and developed a separate program for the older ones, whom we called "Seniors" and who ranged in age from fourteen to eighteen. We began as a coeducational program, although the population was always predominantly male. The younger students were scheduled between breakfast and lunch for a period of tutoring, an instructional swim, art, and horseback riding. After lunch they had a study period on the front porch, or, for the very youngest, a rest period in their cabins. At three o'clock they went for a free swim, and from four to six-thirty a second study period on the front porch. Between supper and bedtime came "evening activities."

The older group, the Seniors, studied all morning except for the period when they were tutored. Those who were tutored before breakfast had an hour off with a choice of activities. After lunch they had art, followed by swimming, another study period, and some free time before supper. After supper they usually had horseback riding in the long summer evenings.

Of course, since we lived out of doors, much depended on the weather, which was often unpredictable. Especially after supper, we would scan the skies and try to decide whether a projected activity could take place. Usually we could manage a game of capture the flag, a scavenger or treasure hunt, softball or soccer, or an evening hike. Evening skinny-dipping was a popular option, as was tennis, once we built the court. Often the youngest group was content to play in the stream, catching crayfish, building dams, or constructing little boats or water wheels.

On one occasion, the evening hikers got lost in the woods. Of course, this was in the days before cell phones. We dispatched search parties, but the night was very dark and they came back reporting no luck. In the morning we notified the police, who began to worry about some sort of foul play. But soon after the police arrived, the contingent marched back into camp singing. They were none the worse for the experience, although the counselors had suffered from the cold, as they had given their outer garments to the campers. Fortunately, they had managed to build a small fire.

We spent the weekdays with the academic program as our main focus, but the weekends were devoted to all the recreational activities we could devise. Every summer we scheduled white-water rafting on the Ohiopyle River for everyone twelve and over. Groups went to the Youghiogheny Dam for water skiing and swimming. Our older students always visited Frank Lloyd Wright's Falling Water. Fayette County Fair was an event that everyone looked forward to; in the early days there were even car races on an adjoining track. We went spelunking at a time when Laurel Caverns was still a wild cave, and exploring was exciting and some-times even hazardous. A favorite place was the Ohiopyle slide—an area where the stream ran down a channel over a series of flat rocks, and counselors and campers alike wore out blue jeans sliding down. There were picnics and cookouts everywhere. Groups went camping overnight, sometimes for the entire weekend. The weekend ended with a candlelight service in the lodge.

Sunday nights we held a regular staff meeting—when necessary, we would also meet during the week. As the camp grew in size, both tutors and counselors submitted a weekly report every Friday. Since these had to be written on 3x5 cards, they were always brief enough for me to have read them before the meeting; accordingly, we could quickly zero in on any camper about whose progress we had concerns.

One of the traditions we established early on was that no adult would ever pass a camper without greeting the student by name, and if possible, following up with some positive comment: e.g. "I heard you learned to canter yesterday," "I really liked the pot you made in art," "Great t-shirt!" "I heard you got up for the first time on water skis," "You have a great smile." Since our staff-student ratio was always one to two, every camper received a lot of positive feedback every day. And they soon reciprocated and would call out our names from yards away—something visitors often commented on.

Over the years we had some wonderful staff. Living and working together for ten summer weeks enabled us to establish some close and lasting friendships. In the evenings we gathered in the lodge, sat by the fire, drank beer—supplied by the camp, as I never wanted young staff to be driving down the mountain at night in search of a bar. Nowadays, of course, such a thing would be quite unthinkable, but the privilege was rarely if ever abused. Sometimes we listened to music: Joan Baez, Peter Paul and Mary, Simon and Garfunkel. When J.C., one of our art teachers, was there he played the piano, a lovely instrument that I had picked up for a hundred dollars and that lasted for years with only occasional tuning. Sometimes a group would go spelunking at Laurel Caverns—in a cave it makes no difference what the outdoor temperature is, and night is as good as day. After the art center was built, a few people would hang out there and experiment with pottery projects. The tennis court was lit at night and often in use. Sometimes the staff went swimming—the pool was a magical place at night, and the water always seemed warmer than in the daytime.

Shirley Kokesh came to us the second summer. I had hired a city girl, Joanne—from Philadelphia, as I remember. She had stayed through the tutor training, but two days before the campers were due to arrive she found a mouse in her cabin. She was gone the following day even before the early morning mail arrived. We held an emergency staff meeting, and I asked if anyone knew anybody who could fill the slot. One of our teachers, Harry, knew of Shirley, who had just graduated at the top of her class from California State Teachers' College (that is California, PA). The next day she came, dressed for the interview as she had been taught and wearing white gloves and a hat. She remembers the interview and claims that I asked her to give the sounds of the short vowels. Apparently, I had a snake wrapped around my neck and all she could think of was "eeek!" Indeed it is possible, as we used to take the large black snakes that sometimes invaded the cabin area and move them to the church property on the other side of the road. They were harmless, but we did not want the campers finding them curled up in their bunks. Shirley taught at Dunnabeck for many years, and, after the death of her mother, we were able to persuade her to join the Kildonan staff, where she eventually headed the elementary program.

Ann Hall drove all the way from Seattle, Washington in a small car. A gifted teacher, she was with us for many summers, and later her daughter Lesley joined her.

Two grandchildren of my mentor Helaine Durbrow, Mark and Van Westervelt, joined the staff. Mark learned to tutor and became, as was his grandmother, an expert on handwriting. Later he went on to teach at Jemicy, a school for dyslexic students in Baltimore, where he became head of the upper school. Van counseled and worked for at least one summer as head counselor. Eventually he went on to a distinguished career in psychology.

Sam Austell, a potter, came to teach art and eventually married Mary Stuart, our riding instructor. There were other camp marriages. Ann Spiegelberg, another riding instructor, married Ken Brown, whom I had hired as business manager. Karen Neilson married Floyd Cerny, and their son, as a toddler, soon became everybody's favorite. He was quick to learn names and called me "Dee-eye-anna." Mark Westervelt married one of our art teachers. Dunnabeck marriages are generally durable.

Dunnabeck was a world of its own, utterly free from distractions. We even created our own time zone. We kept standard time, so that it was light when we wanted to do our early morning trail rides and tutoring sessions and dark when it was time to put the campers to bed. If some morning the cook was late in arriving and breakfast delayed, we simply - re-set the time, synchronized our watches, and put them back later that evening. Occasionally there were problems. We had to drive to Pittsburgh airport to make a flight and forgot to change to what we called "outside

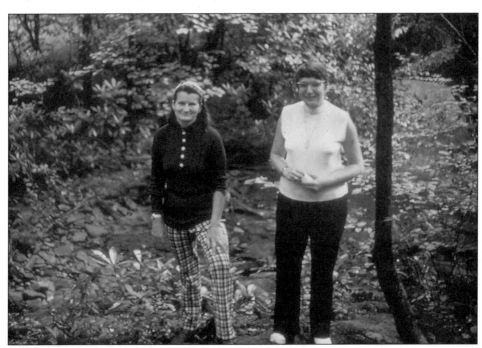

With Shirley Kokesh, doing some planning.

time" as opposed to "Dunnabeck time." I regret to say that over the years, we missed more than one flight. Moreover, during the summer we were generally out of touch with world events. We had no newspapers, and I did not permit radios, for fear that some child might be upset at the news. The only time we ever watched TV was on the occasion of the first moon landing, when we set up a tiny rented black-and-white set on the mantelpiece in the lodge.

Parents visited the third weekend—most of them stayed at the Summit Hotel nearby. We eventually allowed them to keep their children out overnight—at first I feared that doing so would lead to bouts of homesickness. At the hotel families swam in the pool, played tennis, golf, and shuffleboard, and enjoyed all the amenities of the resort hotel. Their children were eager to take them to the slide in Ohiopyle, many of them visited Falling Water, and, once it became commercialized, Laurel Caverns. After Parents' Weekend, we had five uninterrupted weeks for instruction.

We tested our students at the beginning and end of the summer and graphed the usually impressive results to be added to the reports parents received. Students who had never learned to read often did so in the eight weeks, and those who had problems with writing and spelling improved greatly. There were several reasons for our success. There were no outside distractions. The tutors were dedicated, carefully trained, and knew exactly what to do. The study periods provided the necessary reinforcement and drill. Tutors had no responsibilities other than the five morning tutoring sessions and supervision of the afternoon study periods—the latter a duty that was rotated. Their weekends and evenings were free. There were no pressures on students other than those that came from the tutorials. The program of activities was designed to capitalize on the innate strengths of the dyslexic: their sense of balance—water skiing and horseback riding—and their creativity—art.

Nowadays teachers of dyslexic students have at their disposal a plethora of materials, especially workbooks. Aside from the *Gillingham Manual* (first the blue paperback and then the red edition), the accompanying card deck, and the Jewel Box, there was *Eye and Ear Fun* (a series of four workbooks), Mildred Plunket's two books, and later on, *Better Work Habits*. We used the *Buckingham-Ayres Spelling Scale* to build up individual spelling packs for each student. I do not remember our having much in the way of phonetic readers. From the beginning, we read real books aloud, with the tutor keeping the place and supplying any word the student could not decode or recognize. Students practiced writing their spelling words ten times each and wrote hundreds of sentences and compositions as soon as they had developed sufficient sentence skills.

Testing was simple. I had been trained by Helene Durbrow and taught that, if one were sufficiently observant, one ought to be able to test a child for fifteen minutes and have enough information to hold a one-hour conference with the parents. It is not the scores that are important, but the nature of the errors. We used the IOTA, a list of words developed by Marion Monroe, who had worked with Dr. Orton. This test included many of the words that are confusing to dyslexic students. We administered the first form of the WRAT (Wechsler Revised Reading Test), the original *Gray Oral Reading Paragraphs*, and the Gates-MacGinitie for vocabulary, comprehension, and speed. We tested spelling almost weekly, using the Buckingham-Ayres because it has eight different forms. We always stressed cursive handwriting and worked hard to establish correct posture, position, and grip, especially in the case of those left-handed students who had developed a hooked position.

Our campers would often make impressive gains over the summer, spend a year in school, and then return to us just at the level where they had left off. Sometimes, they even lost ground over the course of the entire school year. This problem increasingly concerned me, and I thought that as soon as my own children were old enough, I would start a school where dyslexic students would be able to learn all year long, because the teaching would be appropriate to their learning style.

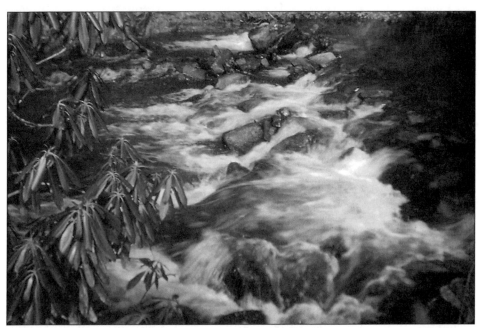

The stream ran the length of the property. For young campers it was a wonderful place in which they played happily for hours, catching crayfish and making dams. Although there was no supervision, some adult was always within earshot.

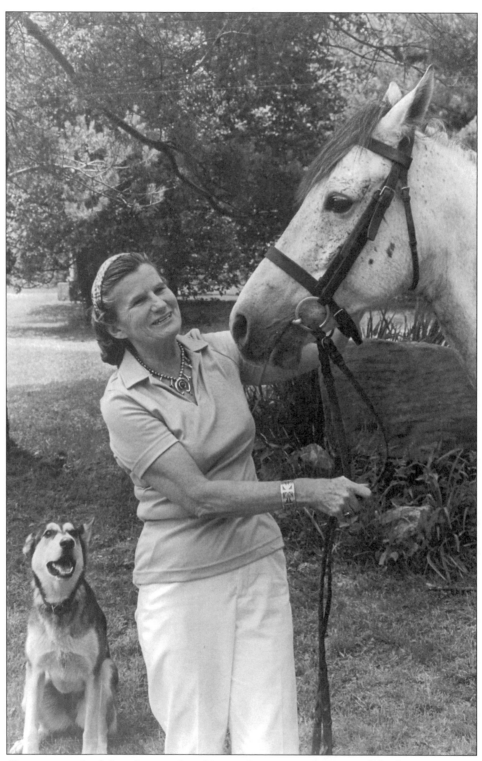

Fen, my wonderful malamute, laughing as I try to reassure one of the horses.

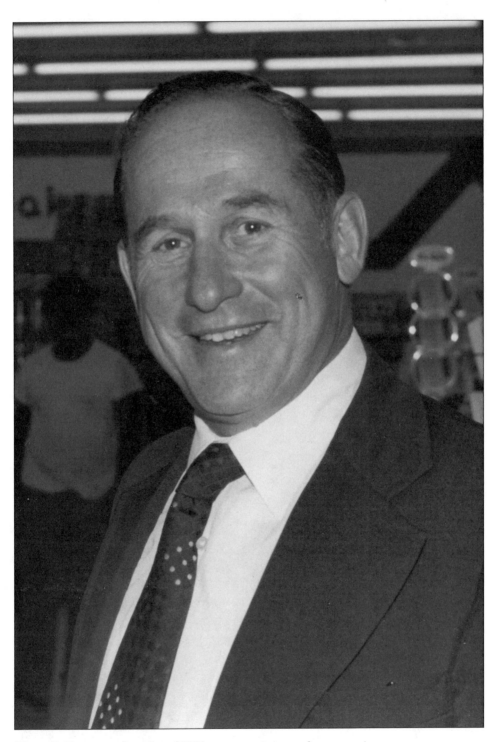

Kurt Goldman, co-founder of Kildonan, continues to be our main support.

~ 5 ~

Kildonan — The Early Years

I always knew that any school I founded would be established as a non-profit organization under the aegis of a board of directors. Dunnabeck was unincorporated and never made money. I also realized that such a school would be dependent on contributions to get started, and, as I later learned, for on-going expenses. Because we had always had a number of students from the Baltimore area—most of them referred by Roger Saunders, a psychologist who specialized in dyslexia—I began looking there. Certainly, there were parents willing to support the project, and, together with some of them, I began driving to Baltimore in search of properties. We found at least one possible piece of land with buildings that would get us started—although in retrospect it was far too small. Then came the question of licensing. I was informed that with my educational background, and my M.A. in philology, I would not be qualified even to teach in Maryland, let alone to run a school. Furthermore, I was informed, the state could never license a school with an unbalanced curriculum and an overemphasis on reading and spelling. Of course, times changed, and at least three schools for dyslexic students, Jemicy, Summit, and Odyssey, flourish there.

Discouraged, I left for the summer and Dunnabeck, where at least I knew I could operate legally. Some years before, I had received a letter from Harrisburg, stating that the authorities had learned that I was operating an illegal school. I had replied that what I was running was a camp, and that kept them quiet for a few years. Eventually, they wrote back informing me that any institution that offered instruction to five or more students was a school, and that they would be sending an inspector to see what we were doing.

In due course the inspector arrived. I had told him in a phone conversation that he might want to know that the program was for dyslexic students. He asked me to spell the word, but when he arrived it was apparent to me that he had not done his homework. As he walked around the camp, he kept commenting, "handsome looking youngsters," and "fine young boys!" Goodness knows what he expected. In any event, I was duly issued a "headmistress's certificate." Ironically, years later after we moved Dunnabeck to New York State, we were informed that the summer program had to be classified as a camp because of the number of activities we offered.

Then came yet another miracle. In the summer of 1968 on Parents' Day in the middle of camp, Kurt Goldman, father of one of the campers, approached me. He said, "Now, about that school that you have talked about wanting to start…you go ahead with your plans, and I will take care of the finances." I was touched and thought to myself, "What a lovely man." And then I promptly forgot about his offer, because I could not imagine that he had meant it. But at the end of the summer, he sought me out, reiterated his offer, and suggested that we go in search of a suitable property. I realized that he was serious. So in the fall we picked up his son, Steven, from his little boarding school in Virginia and drove along the James River in Virginia looking at real estate. There were some lovely mansions, either in various stages of decay or ostentatiously remodeled— I retain a memory of one place with gold-plated faucets in the bathrooms.

Some time later he called to say that he had found something that seemed like a good possibility. It was located in Stockton, a small town on the Delaware, and consisted of several buildings situated on about sixty-five acres of open fields and woodlands. The main building had been used by a summer program, Summerfield, which would continue in operation when we vacated the place and went to Dunnabeck for the summer. There was adequate dormitory space, a dining room and kitchen, several classrooms, and an attractive front space for offices. Other buildings included what had been a carriage house with four small rooms and a three-story stone house, the ground floor of which became our rec room with pool table and snack bar, and the upper two floors of which became my living space. A magnificent stone barn (it had been built originally for an artist who made stained glass windows) adjoining a walled boxwood garden became the art center, and, later on, the emergency dining room. There were two stables and paddocks for our horses—Summerfield had a riding program. And there was a long, low building that had been a chicken coop and that we eventually remodeled into tutoring rooms. This was to be our school for eleven years.

Unlike Maryland, Pennsylvania welcomed our school. Since I was already running what they deemed to be a school, there was no trouble with my certification. We opened with twelve students, but by Christmas we had almost twice that number.

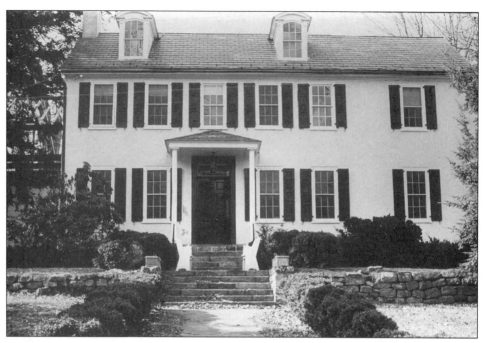

The main house of our Solebury campus.

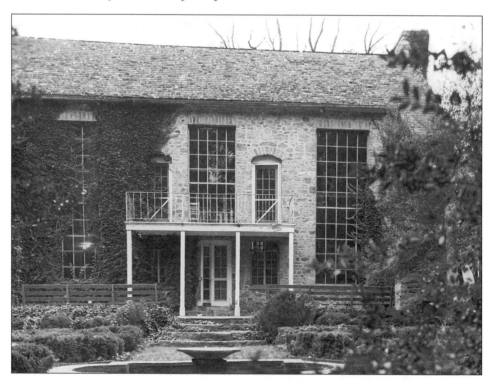

The magnificent stone barn that served as an art room and as a dining room for part of our last year in Pennsylvania.

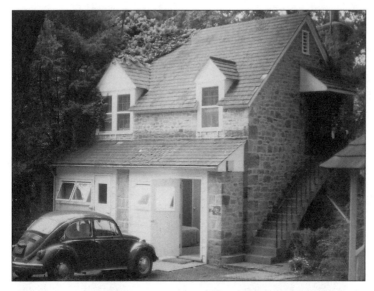

The carriage house, where the older students lived.

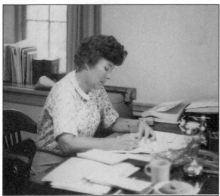

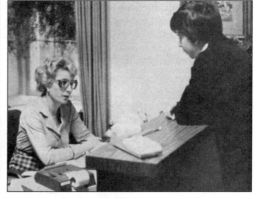

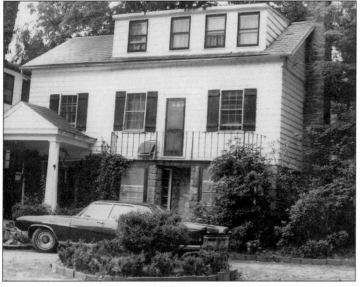

Above: Joan Goldman volunteered her services as our first secretary and bookkeeper until we found Renata Hermes, on right advising a student.

Left: The rec room was down-stairs and my living quarters upstairs.

We knew of schools that served a dyslexic population where the curriculum was confined to the teaching of reading, writing, and arithmetic. I did not want to follow that model. Accordingly, with my colleagues, I began to work out a curriculum that would include history and geography, science, and literature. The history was to focus on concepts more than on facts and dates. Science, as much as possible a hands-on subject, would involve the environment. Literature would afford an opportunity to expose students to books that, in most cases, they would not have been able to tackle on their own. I was determined to have our students read real books rather than anthologies of excerpts. Subject matter classes were taught without textbooks, and because all the work had to be done within the class periods, students were free to concentrate on math and language assignments during their study periods. I expected to prepare most students to be able to move on in two years; accordingly, we designed two-year curricula for each level.

Our early staff was recruited from teachers who had worked at Dunnabeck. Penny van Hoover took charge of the five girls. Dell Sherk taught science, and later the Allens, Bruce and Terry, taught history, mathematics and literature. Lew Fisher taught literature. I taught literature and algebra. All of us tutored, as we wanted to continue the daily one-on-one tutorials that had been the backbone of the summer program. Our students were to range in age from eight to nineteen. We divided them into groups for their classes: Juniors, Middlers, and later Upper Middlers, and Seniors.

Always believing that our population would be a migrant one and that our students would move on once their skills were strong enough, we adopted flying geese as our symbol. The campus was situated on a flyway, and we watched them every spring and fall. When many years later we moved to New York State, again we watched the geese migrating; thus our logo became a link between the two campuses. I asked students whether they wanted a motto in Latin or in English—not surprisingly they asked for English. Our motto became "in quietness and in confidence" taken from the Biblical *Isaiah 30:15*, "in returning and rest shall ye be saved; in quietness and in confidence shall be your strength."

The first year we had an art program, and the second year I told students we could afford to add either music or woodshop. Overwhelmingly, they voted for woodshop. Later attempts to add music were rarely successful. Most students had difficulty singing in tune and reading music. There were exceptions; Jim Mosca played the guitar and went on to a career in fusion jazz.

Gradually the school took advantage of the craftsmen in nearby

New Hope and Peddlars' Village. At various times we were able to offer leatherworking, ceramics, stained glass, and more ambitious woodworking. These activities were popular, in part because they were held off campus.

As we had no gym, our stress was on individual sports. Everybody learned to ride. We engaged in various track and field events in the spring. As the school grew in size, we added soccer and, in the last years, lacrosse—then a new sport that our Baltimore students brought to the campus. In the winter there was skiing and ice-skating, and in the spring tubing and rafting on the Delaware River. I had learned to scuba dive in the Virgin Islands while on vacation there with my children, and had become intrigued with the possibilities of that sport. We were fortunate to find a pair of competent instructors in nearby Princeton. Our students had to make their open-water dives in a nearby quarry, wearing full wet suits because the water was ice cold. Most of our older students earned their PADI certification. We also developed a rock-climbing program.

The second or third winter we had a snowfall followed by a day of rain, which then froze into a hard glaze. Students were able to ice skate all over the campus. I took some groups of students skiing, first at Belle Mountain, then at Camelback or Bear Mountain. In vain I tried to persuade the skaters to join us, but they refused, preferring to enjoy the skating. Finally the sheet of ice that had covered the campus melted, and they joined us for one of the last ski days of the season. At the end of the day two of them came up and said that it was the best thing they had done in their lives. I said, "Well, I did try to tell you." One of them said, "You should have made us do it!" And from then on, winter skiing became mandatory. I don't know when we first settled on Thursday as our ski day, but I do remember my reasoning. Weekends were too crowded, as was Friday. On Mondays the slopes, worn down by the weekend crowd, were often in poor shape. But by Thursday, in anticipation of the weekend crowd, the slopes had to be groomed. Once everybody had learned to ski, we were ready for our ski week. We took the younger students to Stratton Mountain and the older group to Killington.

During the ski season, we held classes on Saturday mornings to make up for the time lost in skiing. During the rest of the year, we used Saturday mornings for work projects around the campus, maintaining the grounds and gardens.

I always kept our camp tradition of sending groups camping on weekends. We also took advantage of theater and museums in New York and of the Macarthur Theater in Princeton. After all, we could be on Broadway in a little over an hour. Many of our students had never

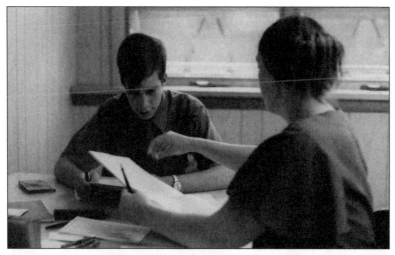

*Jane Unger
tutoring.*

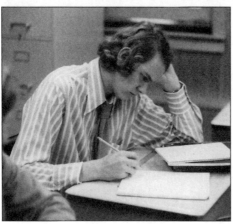

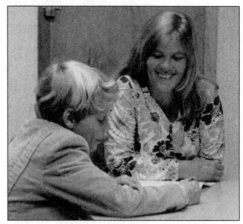

*Pictured above: (left) Charlie Kilgore,
son of one of our trustees, struggling
with an algebra problem. (Right) Penny
van Hover tutoring a young student.
No wonder Scott Crawford decided to
marry her on the strength of this photo!*

*Right: At that time we had some very
young boarding students. Some of them
came from as far away as Vancouver,
B.C.*

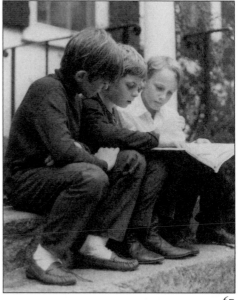

67

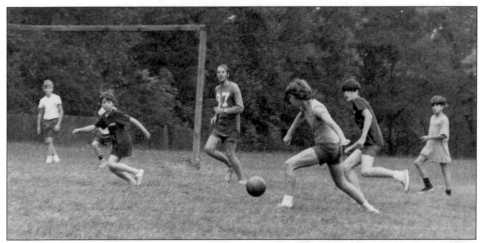

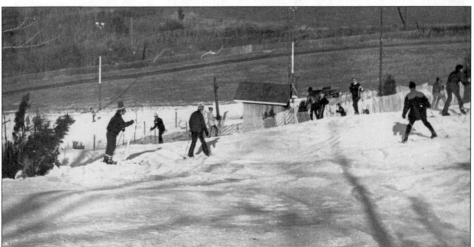

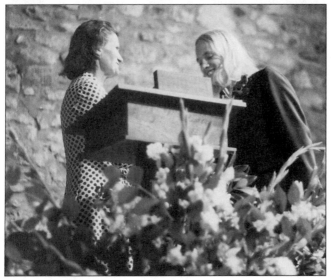

Top: Tom Unger
coaching soccer.

Center: Belle Mountain,
where our students
began their skiing. They
nicknamed it Belle
Bump because of its size.

Left: Graduation in the
boxwood garden in front
of the stone barn. I am
awarding a diploma to
Malcolm Bell-Irving.

experienced the thrill of live theater before. When we went to see *One Flew over the Cuckoo's Nest*, a student laughed so loudly that I thought we might be asked to leave the theater. In *Equus*, during the scene where the girl takes off her clothes, students turned to gauge my reaction. As it happened, I was quite unfazed because I had already seen the production and deemed it appropriate.

Our trustees continued to be wonderfully generous and supportive. Kurt Goldman, the Chairman of our Board, assumed supervision of the finances of the school. He and his associate, Sal di Bianca, came every Saturday night to take over the kitchen and make pizza (then more of a novelty than it is now) for the entire group. His wife, Joan, ran the office, answering the phone and coping with routine correspondence. Kurt's mother, Marie, was always available to me when I needed to sit and talk over a cup of tea. She reminded me of my beloved great-grandmother, Eleanor Rawnsley, and her advice was always sage. Since budgeting and financial planning has never been a skill, nor even an interest of mine, the accounts and bills were managed at the office of Johanna Farms, the dairy production business that the Goldman family owned. Eventually we hired Renata Hermes as accountant and secretary, and she kept meticulous records until we moved the school to Amenia, New York.

My abiding passion was—and still is—teaching, and I was never particularly good at administration. My role models—Robert Grinham at Ruzawi, Frank Barger at Sidwell, and Carol Preston at Potomac were all autocrats. I was better at starting the school than I was at running it. In retrospect, I should have had more training. We ran into problems with our older girls, who would manage to make their way into the boys' rooms late at night, among other things. After a couple of years of experimenting with co-education, we decided to become an all-boys school. This was not to change until many years later, when we had the facilities to accommodate both sexes. In part owing to my naivete and lack of experience, I tended to be far too trusting of our boys. We let them roam the countryside, and once when a couple of them came back late, red-faced and giggling, I did not know enough to suspect that they had been smoking marijuana. I foolishly allowed one student, who was a hunter, to bring a gun to school. We allowed four of them to camp out overnight unsupervised, but when I happened by the campsite the next morning, I found it littered with beer bottles. Our Board felt that while I should continue as Director of Education, the school needed a headmaster. A succession of three men followed. Despite the care the Board took in interviewing and selecting, all three had serious flaws, and were not helped by the fact that I was quick to undermine their authority. It was not until we moved to

Amenia that I became better able to share decision-making.

The faculty continued to grow and the curriculum to evolve and expand. Jane and Tom Unger joined us. Jane had a background in Latin, and was probably the most gifted tutor we ever trained. Tragically, she developed multiple sclerosis at an early age. Tom went on to head the Language Training Department at Solebury School. Scott Crawford taught both mathematics and English, and helped to develop the sports program. On his first day sitting in the faculty room, he saw a picture of Penny van Hoover in the yearbook and said to my daughter Sheila, "That is the woman I will marry." He did, and they are still happily married. During the initial interview process I asked him if he knew how to ski. Scott assured me that he had learned to ski in Scotland. But the first day of the ski season he fell at my feet on the beginner slope. I was surprised, and when he did it again, I became increasingly suspicious. Some years later he confessed that he had lied, because he was confident that, fine athlete that he was—he had set a track record at the University of Pennsylvania—he would pick up the skill over the Christmas break, spending his entire year-end paycheck on instruction.

My son Christopher tutored, as did his young wife, Kathy Gadway. Peter Moses became one of our most imaginative history teachers. He frequently appeared in class in the costume of whatever period of history he was teaching. Once I was momentarily startled in the faculty room when I turned around to see a Zulu warrior, wearing little but a loincloth and carrying a menacing staff. Neil Torgeson expanded the science curriculum to include a study of wind and solar power. After he left us, he founded a solar-power company of his own. He also instituted a series of what we called "habitat" trips, a certain number of which became one of our graduation requirements. Students spent a day in the Pine Barrens, at a winter beach, at the Delaware Water Gap, on a mountain ridge, or by a lake, and were taught to observe everything—the sky, the wind direction, and the flora and fauna that thrived there. At the end of the day they had to write up their observations. It was our hope that they would take this skill with them and become more observant of their environment wherever they were. In the spring when the shad run in the Delaware River, the science classes went to watch the fishermen and brought back enough fish to feed everybody.

~ 6 ~

Creativity and Ingenuity

During the early Dunnabeck years, we had ample opportunity to learn about the characteristics of the dyslexic mind, one of which is ingenuity, and with it, the ability to come up with new ideas and to solve problems in a novel way. Some of the incidents that follow reflect this.

During the rainy summers in the Alleghenies when we could think of absolutely nothing to do with our charges, we took them to the Summit Hotel to play in the game room. I received a complaint from the management that our campers were unlocking the machines and removing the money. When I confronted the culprit, he was quick to confess. "But," he said, "it isn't really stealing. We always put the money back into the machine." Of course, I had a different point of view. That was the summer of the gas shortage, and we had a lock on the tank of our van. Someone lost the key. I approached our locksmith student, and asked him: could he possibly? He took another key from his collection, filed it down, and handed it to me, saying, "I think you will find this works." And it did. Later, he remarked, "Diana, what do you do about having a talent that can get you into trouble?"

Berry Dixon had been one of our students, and one summer we hired him as a counselor. He was in charge of the youngest campers. I always felt that American children had no fixed bedtimes and often did not get sufficient sleep. Our camp day, replete with activities, was strenuous, and unless the children were well rested they would not be able to take advantage of the tutorials that were our *raison d'etre*; accordingly, an after-lunch nap was built into the program. When Berry took over, his charges always went to sleep and had to be awakened for their three o'clock swim. This was in the seventies, and I became a little suspicious and asked him just what he was doing to these children. "It is simple," he said. "I observe them when they are asleep at night and see in what positions they are lying. When rest period comes, I make them lie in those positions and they fall asleep. Isn't that what everybody does?" I have yet to meet a parent to whom this idea has ever occurred.

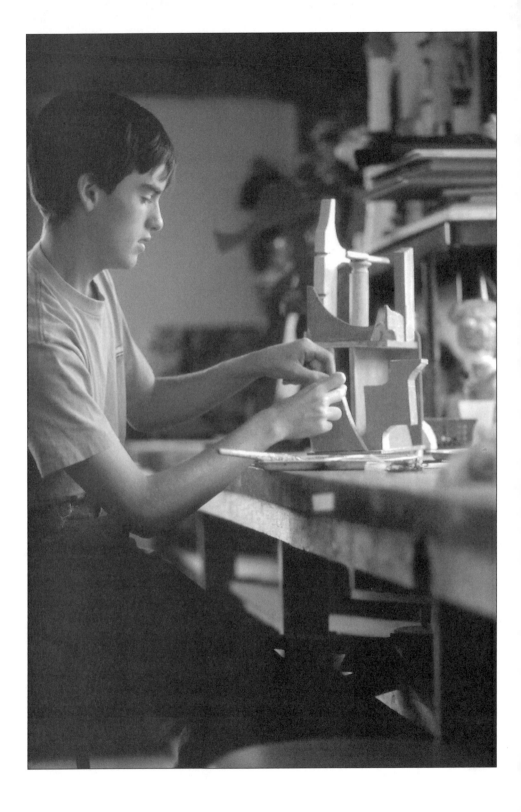

The freezer in which we stored ice cream was in a back room of the barn. The door was locked, but there was a gap between the wall and the rafters. When the cook started complaining that her ice cream supply was being raided, I at first accused the staff. But we found that some of our students were sneaking out at night and climbing over the wall. I had to have some heavy wire mesh nailed across it. I also installed a lock on the freezer as an extra precaution. When we started the school, some students actually tunneled through a wall on the stairway to find their way into the kitchen. When we moved the campus to Amenia, George Vosburg, our first headmaster, at that time new to our population but not to the campus, remarked, "Locks that we have had for years just do not seem to be effective any longer."

During the first couple of years in Amenia, we were unable to afford proper fencing, with the result that our horses occasionally escaped. This was always something of an emergency, and we were afraid they would wander onto the highway and cause accidents. About six of the horses got out one evening at dusk. Betsy, the headmaster's dyslexic daughter, and I set off to find them. Meanwhile, some of the guys were loading buckets of grain and halters into the truck and preparing to follow us. Betsy and I found the horses grazing peacefully on a hillside, but we worried that when the truck came they would be spooked and take off. As we stood petting them, I remarked, "If we just had a piece of rope or something, we could secure the ringleaders and the rest would stay. But we are not even wearing belts." Without hesitating a moment, Betsy replied, "But Diana, we do have our bras." So there in the dark we took off our shirts and used our bras as makeshift halters. The crew in the truck was amazed.

Once I returned to the campus long past midnight. To my surprise, the lights were on in the stone barn. When I investigated, I found a wild game in progress. In imitation of the movie "Rollerball" that they had seen recently, the students had padded themselves with lacrosse and ski gear, complete with goggles, and were engaged in a wild game of roller ball. So engrossed were they that they were slow to notice me standing in the doorway. When they did, I merely remarked, "Why don't you all just go to bed and get some sleep."

In Pennsylvania, when the drinking age was still eighteen, I foiled their attempts to buy liquor by taking Polaroid shots of the seniors and giving them to the owner of the liquor store across the bridge. Over the years, they made various attempts to grow marijuana. At Cricket Hill, where we later moved our Seniors, there was a small bed close to a water source where I found young plants growing amidst the lettuce I had sown. Once, on an unexpected visit to a student room, I saw a container of seeds on his desk. In answer to my question, Paul Gardner said, "That? That's just birdseed. Don't you know that people eat it as a snack? It is quite popular these days." Nevertheless, I pocketed his supply, but there must have been more of it because, as I later found out, they had sown it between the rows of corn in a nearby farm. In the fall when they came back to school to harvest it, they were disappointed. The plants were puny, and there was barely enough for a single joint.

We never did manage to discover who had tapped into the phone line or who had removed all the valuable copper piping from the chicken coop. And there were other unsolved mysteries. I never did find out who had put a very dead mouse into the toe of my ski boot, but the scream I let out in the lodge as I pulled it out, thinking it was just one of those silk socks, must have afforded great satisfaction.

One of our spring sports was track, and students who participated were allowed to go off running by themselves, or in groups of two or three. One pair took advantage of this option, and returned every afternoon convincingly drenched in sweat. On a whim, I happened to be doing a little exploring in the woods when I came across a beautifully constructed underground hideout. It was even carpeted, and there were tins and bottles of various contraband material and food. It was roofed with planks, and had apparently been camouflaged with a layer of earth and leaves. So, this was how a pair of students had used their sports period!

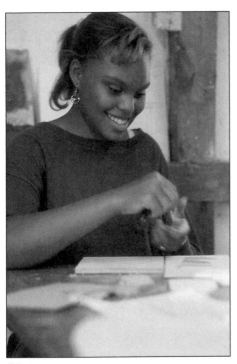 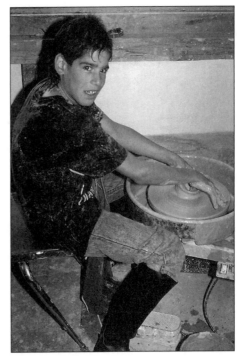

At Kildonan, as at most boarding schools, weekends are always something of a challenge. During the weekdays, all students are accounted for at all times. Keeping students occupied on Saturday and Sunday is more difficult—we know what the devil finds for idle hands. Our routine was to devote Saturday mornings to work projects on campus, and to do those things for which our maintenance crew never had time and for which we could not afford to hire outside help. One fall morning I decided to have the older students plant bulbs, of which I had purchased an ample supply. I got them started, and went off to spend the rest of the morning raking leaves with the younger group. At lunch that day, one of the older students commented that he had never planted anything except a light bulb and had been uncertain as to which way up to plant them. In answer to my question, he said, "I put most of them in with the pointed side down because they seemed to go in more easily that way." I was not too worried because I knew that bulbs have the ability to turn themselves. All through the winter from time to time the bulb planters would ask, "When do you think our bulbs will be coming up," or look at me and say, "I just can't wait to see our bulbs in the spring." A passionate gardener myself, I was delighted to think of these young lads beginning to develop what would perhaps become a life-long interest in horticulture.

Spring came. One morning I was teaching my algebra class when John, our maintenance man, interrupted me. He said, "I need to talk to you." "John," I said, "couldn't it wait till recess?" "I don't think so," he replied. So I assigned the homework, told my students to start on it if I did not return, and followed John out of the building. "Diana," he said, "you have got to see what is coming up right by the front entrance to the school." Well, the crocuses spelled the f___ word, and the daffodils the sh___ word—perfectly and clearly spelled out. I instructed John to do a bit of replanting and, pondering the perils of the creative dyslexic mind, returned to my class,

On the one hand, creativity is a wonderful advantage. Edison and Einstein are always cited as the classic examples (role models for the dyslexic that I deplore, for reasons to be discussed later in this book). Linda Edmark, the Texas gal who invented the topsy tail, is, I think, a more legitimate example. Severely dyslexic, she wondered whether she could turn a ponytail inside out. She fiddled about with a toothbrush and a rubber band and a pencil and a paper clip. Then, because she was a knitter, she had the bright idea of cutting a circular knitting needle in half, and she had her little gadget—it looks rather like a bubble blower. At first she and her maid sat at the kitchen table stuffing envelopes and opening envelopes with ten-dollar bills in them. Then she used her savings, got a loan from the bank, and went commercial. When last heard of, she had made thirty-two million dollars. In one interview she said, "I used to think of my dyslexia as a curse. Now I consider it a blessing, for without it I never could have become an inventor."

On the other hand, as is readily apparent from some of the examples above, a dyslexic mind is a great asset to a criminal. Not only the ingenuity, but the innate charm, keen attention to detail, and the acting ability are designed for success in the underworld. And, of course, those who have remained illiterate and unable to find employment are in double jeopardy. Later on, I was to have an opportunity to learn more about this first-hand. Roger Saunders, my Baltimore psychologist friend, received a letter from an inmate in Sullivan County's maximum-security prison. He wanted to learn to read and wondered whether a teacher could be found who would come to him. Roger passed the letter on to me. At the time, I was in temporary retirement from Kildonan and had nothing particular to do. So, for about a year and a half I drove twice a week, making the two-hundred-mile round trip to the prison in Fallsburg. The building was state-of-the-art, and it took me a while to become accustomed to the array of security measures—I had to pass through seven locked doors to get to the teaching area. Polly Ashe, who was to become my friend, was helpful at initiating me into procedures and at making me welcome. I taught a small group of men—as I recall there were six or seven of them. All of them were almost totally illiterate. They were black, Hispanic, and one was Chinese. I wondered how they would react to a white teacher. I concentrated on two things that I thought might save me: I exaggerated my British accent and I worked at being a grandmotherly figure. I established a first-name basis. And it worked. The first day I realized that I would have to teach them something if I was going to be able to hold them. They all needed money, and the system was such that they could earn more by doing janitorial work around the prison than by attending classes and learning to read. Since they evidently knew consonant sounds and letter names, I decided to begin with the silent-e principle. I had them read words such as *home, late, safe, hope,* and *mine.* As he read these words, one of them, José, became increasingly agitated and his voice more and more high-pitched. "It's okay, José," I said. You are doing fine." He stood up, and practically shouted, "You don't understand. Nobody understands." I barely had time to wonder what on earth to do—call Security for help?— when he finished, "It is the first time in my life that I have ever read words." He did learn to read in the time I spent there. Another memorable student was a Chinese, the youngest member of the group. He had been picked up almost straight off the boat from China; probably, Polly told me, because of involvement with a New York gang. He told me that when he was first taken to his cell, he thought it must be the bathroom. I think he was probably a bright student in China, accustomed to doing well. He was my star pupil, until one day I taught the syllabication rule that involves knowing vowel length. He quickly became frustrated, for how was he to know whether the word was ca-bin or cab-in, and laid his head down on the desk and kept it there for the rest of the class. I did not disturb him. On another occasion—in those days they were allowed a cigarette break—I watched his confusion as a fellow inmate asked him for a light. He pointed to the nearest lighting fixture and could not understand why the group laughed at him. One of my more treasured possessions is a letter he wrote me after I had left. It was in Chinese, and I had to take it to the nearby Chinese restaurant for translation. It was a touching thank-you note, explaining what a difference I had made to his life by caring about him. One particularly charming inmate was removed from the group. I had noticed that he liked to sit next to me. What he had been doing was attaching a little mirror to the top of his shoe and moving it around so as to be able to look up my skirt. He cannot have had much satisfaction—my skirt was long and I wore a slip. Some days later, I passed him in the hallway, and he said he was sorry, and I told him that I was not angry.

They loved being read to. I selected *Charlotte's Web* as our first book, for I thought, who can resist that first sentence, '*Where's Pa going with that axe?' asked Fern.*" The scene in which Wilbur escapes and is being chased by everybody particularly delighted the inmates in my class. The prison had a splendid library full of law books, but nothing for beginning readers. I spoke to the librarian and suggested he acquire a selection of children's literature. He replied that nobody would ever take them out. So, with my own money I brought in a selection—*Curious George* books, and as many of the *Boxcar Children* series as I could find. Polly Ashe's group wanted them too, and we kept having to find more. One inmate remarked, "We had these when I was at school, but I could never read them and now I can." I brought in some of Langston Hughes' poems, and they asked for copies, saying that they wanted to send them to people they loved. Polly and I had been encouraging the men to read in the evenings in their cells, but they often became frustrated and gave up when they came across a word they could not decode. I bought a couple of Franklin Speak and Spell machines, so that they would be able to punch in the words and hear them—of course, we had to get permission from Security to do this. Later, the prison bought more. One day I asked them to write about what their dreams were, what they would do when (not if) they were ever released.

One inmate wrote a wonderful description that, alas, I no longer have, of a future. It would begin with the selling of hot chestnuts on the street, and would expand into a tiny store with hotdogs, pickles, candy, and coffee, and would be a place where all his friends would come to hang out.

Were they dyslexic? I think so. Bright as they were, they would otherwise surely have picked up at least rudimentary reading skills. Certainly they showed all the reversals, such as the b/d confusion that plague the dyslexic. And their ingenuity was obvious.

Half-way through the experience, I came to the conclusion that the best way of helping the illiterate population in jails was to train those who were literate to act as tutors. I started with a fairly large group, and even though most of them dropped out after a couple of sessions, I was able to give the rest of them the sort of training we were giving our new tutors at Dunnabeck and Kildonan. By the time I left, they were already beginning to tutor.

The prison experience was a valuable one. It left me with two things: a lifelong aversion to the death penalty and a realization of the connection between illiteracy and recidivism, and, of course, of the importance of early intervention and remediation that would prevent dyslexics from ending up in a life of crime.

Roger Saunders, with some others, had founded a program in Baltimore called MAYDAY, that was involved in persuading judges to sentence young delinquents to learn to read. They were given forty lessons by a trained volunteer tutor. The only real expense was in the hiring of a psychologist to do the initial screening to establish their ability to benefit from the program, and the salary of the teacher who would do the training and supervise the teachers. They also had to have an office manned by a volunteer to coordinate the program. They raised the necessary funds by appealing to local businesses. MAYDAY is a success, and has the statistics to prove it. I longed to be able to establish something similar in nearby Poughkeepsie, and attempted to do so. The county supervisor was interested, and I had several meetings with her and with some other people. But then came elections that brought a change of regime, and I was unable to pursue the project, much to my regret.

~ 7 ~

We Move

The school continued to grow, and our quarters in Stockton to become increasingly crowded. By the terms of our lease, there were limits to our ability to expand. Our population of young boys was increasing. Accordingly, while I was away running Dunnabeck, Kurt Goldman arranged for some additional dorm space. I had left with a plan that involved four separate rooms, but when I returned at the end of the summer, I found the planned partitions eliminated, and one large European style dormitory room that was to house our ten students. Needless to say, bedtime became a huge problem. Our Upper Middlers were in a room with four bunk beds, but they were older and easier to settle down at night. Then, one summer, we found we had enrolled too many students for the available space. With the help of my son Christopher, who had taken a course in building construction, we set up partitions in the dining room and converted that space into sleeping quarters before school opened. Meals for the fall term were in the Stone Barn, carried over in insulated containers. As the weather became cooler, we built huge fires in the fireplace and everybody wore sweaters. But by the end of the fall term, it was too cold to continue.

Through the generosity of a local real estate agent, we were able to rent Cricket Hill, a lovely Bucks County style stone house about three miles away on the other side of the Delaware. Because the house was due for remodeling, she was willing to have teenagers living there. I decided to take the oldest group of boys—there were ten of them—and move them onto the Cricket Hill campus. I explained that we would eat supper and breakfast there, and that they would have to take turns cooking and washing up. At first, they protested and suggested that I should have taken the younger students. But after a few days, they loved it. In the beginning, they wanted my help in preparing the evening meals, but soon they took pride in doing the cooking unsupervised. There were several amusing incidents. One of the assigned cooks, in response to complaints about the baked potatoes, said, "Well, I did not want them to cook so long that they would be hard." One ski day we had left Richard Zirinsky—exempt from skiing because of his lack of balance—in charge, and I had instructed him to cook the rice in some leftover chicken stock. But when he went to begin the process, the refrigerated stock had jelled. Worried at the prospect of being faced by hungry returning skiers, he called his mother for advice. "Silly," she said, "it's just like chicken aspic. It will melt when you heat it." Evening study hall was either in their rooms or in the living area. I did some random supervision. Once I wandered into a student room and on impulse picked up a blanket only to discover a contraband TV. The student was quick to protest that he had been studying and was not watching it. But I leaned down, touched it and asked, "Then why is it warm?" He lost his room study privileges.

Our Cricket Hill lease was just for half a year, and we had to find new quarters for the school. Elizabeth Mills, known as Leisket, was the indefatigable chair of our Board, and she embarked on a search. At one point she asked me how I felt about a merger. This was a period when many schools were in search of solutions to their falling enrollment problems. I told her that this would not be an acceptable solution—for there would always be their students and we would become "those kids." We did some traveling. I remember an orphanage, one enormous building with rows of little sinks in the bathrooms. I felt strongly that our energetic students could not survive cooped up in one building. We came close to settling on Fox Hollow, the former Edith Wharton place. It was a glorious situation, and I fell in love with the stables, but negotiations broke down. Then, through Leisket's connections with NAIS, the National Association of Independent Schools, we found the perfect place.

Barlow School had been a type of alternative school for bright but troubled adolescents, and had been unable to attract a sufficient number of students to survive. Thanks to the skilled negotiation of Leisket and Kurt Goldman, we were able to buy the 460-acre property with all the buildings on incredibly reasonable terms. We paid off some of their debts and took on a three-hundred-thousand-dollar, interest-free mortgage.

I still remember our first sight of the campus. As we drove along Perry's Corners Road the view opened up. The sun was shining on green playing fields and a pond. The road turned towards the school buildings, and behind them the land sloped upward into the hillside. The facility was more than adequate for our needs. There were several dormitories, which we named for famous dyslexics: Amy Lowell, Winston Churchill, Thomas Edison, Hans Christian Andersen, Woodrow Wilson, Albert Einstein, and Leonardo da Vinci. The schoolhouse, built in the style of a barn, the library, and the art center were all at the bottom of the hill. The dining room and dormitories were on top of the hill, so that our students got plenty of exercise walking up and down.

The Barlow headmaster, George Vosburg, and his wife Melissa agreed to stay on. I liked them immediately, and the Board arranged that George would be our new headmaster, and I would be Director of Education. This arrangement survived for several happy years. Both were young and energetic. George knew nothing about dyslexia even though his daughter Betsy was dyslexic, but he was quick to learn. Melissa learned to tutor and organized the weekend activities, instituting a fine program that enabled every student to get off campus for at least one day. Several other Barlow School teachers stayed on, including Pony Simon, who taught art history, and Virginia Haaland, who taught English. The cook, Sylvia Schultz, was to be with us for over twenty years; Harold "Smitty" Smith worked in the maintenance crew until his retirement, and Lionel Summers until his death. Peg Fanelli was our first bookkeeper, and Carol Kapell the school secretary. At the end of the first year, we were singularly lucky in finding Ann Still as business manager, a position she still holds at the time of this writing.

At the beginning of our first year in Amenia, we hired three teachers who were destined to remain with us for many years. Joan Worswick became a fine tutor, working especially successfully with the more severely dyslexic students. Audrey Walker tutored and taught literature in her time at Kildonan. Both retired after 20 years of service. After her retirement, Audrey became our most valued substitute teacher; I am always relieved when she is available to replace me during my trips to conferences and meetings. Finally, Katherine Schantz, gifted with superb clinical teaching skills, tutored for three years, running the language training program during the summers. She then left us for Harvard and returned as our Academic Dean, eventually becoming Associate Head. She went on to become head of Delaware Valley Friends, a Quaker school for students with learning difficulties in Philadelphia.

When the Vosburgs left, Leisket led another search committee. Of all the candidates who made it to the end of the selection process, Ron Wilson was the most promising. He was married to an attractive and intelligent wife, Bonnie. They had no children at that point. I agreed that he was the best candidate and was delighted when he accepted the position. Over the years, he has demonstrated the consistent leadership skills that I never mastered, and has enabled the school to grow beyond my fondest dreams. Now Ron has two wonderful little boys of his own, both of whom are avid soccer and ice hockey players. I have loved working

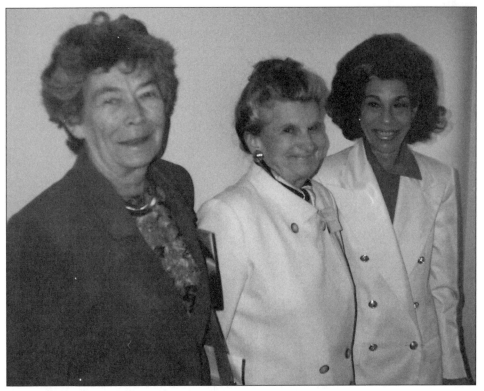

Leisket Mills, our indefatigable Board Chair, with me and Barbara Hoffman, wife of Eli, another faithful trustee.

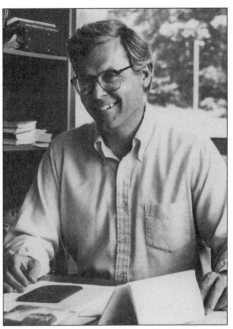

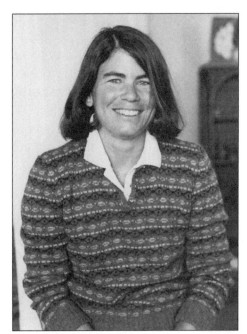

George and Melissa Vosburgh

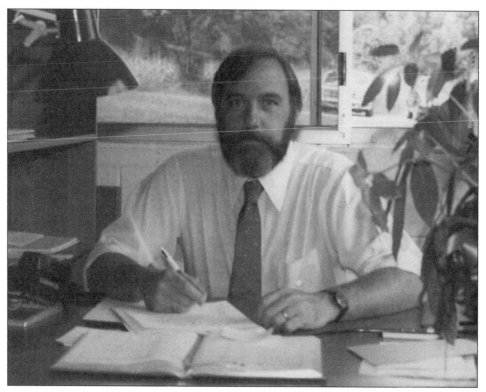

Ron Wilson, taken before he had been aged by the rigors of heading Kildonan.

with him and increasingly appreciate the depth of his compassion and caring for students. Over the years, he has become strong and forceful in dealing with aberrant faculty, and in solving difficult and sensitive personnel and parent problems. Bonnie is an excellent tutor, and now does an outstanding job as Director of Admissions.

For some years I had tried to persuade Shirley Kokesh to come to Kildonan, but she wanted to stay where she could care for her mother. After her mother died, Shirley joined the faculty. The educational climate had changed, and it was difficult for us to lure young children to boarding school. On the other hand, we had learned from experience—and now there is a massive amount of research to support this idea—that the earlier one can intervene, the greater the chances for success. At first we had a small group in a room in the art center under the direction of Christine Killmer. In 1998, thanks to the generosity of our trustees, we were able to build an Elementary Learning Center. Shirley was involved in designing the building and insisted that there be lots of windows—even the individual tutoring rooms needed windows—wide hallways, and student bathrooms attached to every classroom. Today, the building accommodates 40 students in grades 2 through 6. Some of them are driven nearly two hours, morning and evening, in order to attend. Because of the long commute so many of them have to make, no homework is ever assigned; independent work has to be completed during the in-school study halls.

Shortly after our move to the Amenia campus, computers became available. I was excited by the possibility and thought that we should invest in the least expensive available. But our trustees, with their usual foresight, wanted to study the matter further and made sure we spent our funds wisely. We ended up with the early Macintosh models. Through the years, we have steadily increased our number of computers; we now have over a hundred, and many students bring their own computers or laptops to school. From the first, we insisted on correct fingering and taught classes in keyboarding. One summer in Pennsylvania, a student had brought a typewriter, and his parents expected him to learn to type over the course of the summer. We searched Uniontown without being able to find a book, and I was forced to improvise. I began by teaching him to type his name, keeping his hands on the home keys and his eyes averted. He learned immediately. Then I began teaching him the alphabet, always having him name each letter aloud as he struck the key and refrain from looking at his hands. He learned the keyboard within a couple of days and was soon able to type fairly rapidly. I had forgotten about this experience until many years later, when we needed to teach our Kildonan students to type.

The advantages of correct keyboarding are manifold. Obviously it is faster than hunt-and-peck, but with correct keyboarding the brain is gradually programmed so that spelling of common words becomes automatic. For most dyslexics, a spell check is a godsend for more complex words. There are many students who in earlier years would have managed college, if only computers had been available to them. I described what we were doing to Bob Hall, the head of the family-owned Educators Publishing Service, and he asked me whether I thought the description of my keyboarding technique could be made into a book. I sat down and wrote the book in a little over a week, and it has enabled thousands of all ages to learn keyboarding. Students who have difficulty in learning in the conventional way, home keys first, followed by keys above and below them, could master the letters in less than half an hour.

Once I went to Jemicy School and offered to demonstrate, if they would provide me with a group of ten-year-olds. When I arrived at the school I observed a boy in the parking lot kicking rocks around. I asked what his problem was, and the teacher said, "He wanted to do it but he is only eight, and you said they had to be ten." Of course I welcomed him into the group. By the time the rest of the students had mastered the alphabet and were having fun spelling out other words, he was more than half-way through the alphabet and doing just fine. Computers are truly "touch-typing," and the finger strength required for old-fashioned type-writers is no longer needed; as soon as students' hands are big enough, they can begin—certainly third grade is not too early. For adults who decide to attend college late in life, keyboarding is a vital asset. Using my book, they can become proficient in a matter of weeks. The problem with allowing students to hunt-and-peck is that they become fairly quick at it, and do not want to slow down and learn correct fingering. At both Kildonan and Dunnabeck, students have to demonstrate proficiency in touch-typing before they are allowed to use a computer for their assign-ments. I recently learned that with correct fingering, carpel tunnel problems are less likely to develop.

Students who dislike writing often change their attitude once they can keyboard. They do enjoy exchanging e-mails with friends and, while they are away from home, even with their parents. The benefits of being able to go online rather than engaging in what, for them, is frustrating library research, is another asset.

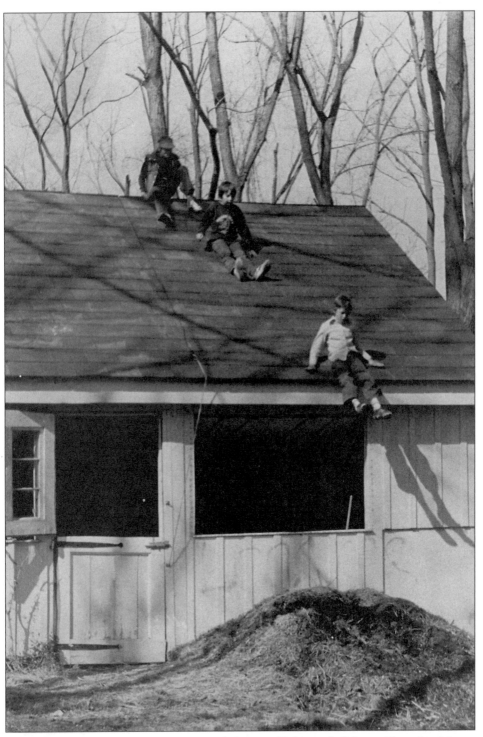

In Pennsylvania, young students enjoyed sliding off the roof of the stable to land in the soft pile of manure below.

~ 8 ~

✣ High Energy ✣

Certainly there does seem to be an overlap between hyperactivity and dyslexia; on the other hand, ADHD is frequently over-diagnosed. We have always had restless and active students in our program. Sometimes the restlessness, accompanied at times by endless yawning during tutorials, is a result of the frustration experienced in the past. Sometimes it disappears as students become more successful in their studies, or as they move through adolescence. I dislike the term hyperactivity and prefer to call it, "high energy." In adult life, as we shall see later, it becomes a tremendous asset. At Kildonan we manage our young students in several ways. During any listening activity, they are allowed to draw and even to play with quiet toys. Elementary students are all scheduled for a period of horseback riding in the middle of the morning. For older students, moving from class to class, often between buildings, seems to help, as does time spent walking up and down the hill. They are often scheduled for an art or a woodworking class in the morning, and are sometimes permitted to draw during lecture portions of classes. The afternoon sports activities provide an outlet for all ages. In the summer program, we schedule tutorials for our younger campers during one of the first two periods right after breakfast.

For some students ritalin, or one of the allied drugs, is a necessity. Even in the tutorials, the difference is immediate and evident; a tutor can tell right away if a student has missed a dose—not only immediate learning, but also retention seems to be affected. Parents are often apprehensive at the prospect of having their children placed on any form of medication. However, recent research on the long-term effects of these drugs supports the idea that there are no ill effects. Moreover, the I.Q.'s of medicated students went up, presumably because they were able to attend better and to absorb information.

Another aspect of the overly active mind seems to be disorganization. Roger Saunders, both dyslexic and disorganized, once remarked, as

I eyed his desk, "Diana, everything I touch just turns to clutter." Teachers are frustrated by the book bag full of loose papers and the three-ring notebooks with all the pages falling out, as well as by messy lockers and desks. Organizing possessions and clothing are other areas of difficulty. At Camperdown Academy students keep a notebook with color-coded sections for every subject. At the end of each class, the teacher instructs students, "File this handout right behind the yellow divider." At Kildonan we provide younger students with eight-pocket folders in which to keep their assignments. In the middle and upper school we are experimenting with a handbook for recording assignments—as yet not entirely satisfactory. Clothing is another matter. When we were at Dunnabeck in Western Pennsylvania, campers had to keep their clothing in a trunk. Sometimes we would help young campers by removing all but a two-day supply, and as they improved, gradually giving them more to organize. Parents of dyslexics should begin when their children are young by teaching them organizational skills.

Louise Clarke, author of *Can't Read Can't Write Can't Talk Too Good Either* (in the original edition the letters in the word *talk* were transposed to read *tlak*, but every librarian in the country promptly corrected it!), discovered to her surprise that her son flourished in the structured environment of Saint Bernard's. Anna Carlson, Director of Academic Advising and Support at New England College, wondered how students raised in a highly structured boarding school would compare with those from public school when they were turned loose in the freedom college offers. She discovered that they did just fine—actually, somewhat better than those whose academic lives had been less structured. Presumably, what happens is that students eventually internalize the structure.

Not only are dyslexics lost in space, but time is also a problem. Once I was observing my friend Ann Vickers tutor a third-grade girl. Towards the end of the lesson the little girl became agitated and said she did not know where to go next. Together, they looked at her schedule. "Well, what day is it today?" Ann asked. "Thursday…Tuesday…no, Wednesday," the child guessed. Actually, it was Monday. Her confusion would have been more understandable had it been the middle of the week, but Monday comes right after the weekend, and ever since kindergarten that child would have gone through exercises that involve the calendar.

Telling time is difficult, and even by adolescence many students are fine with digital watches but cannot always tell time on an analog clock; naturally, this is a source of embarrassment that they try to conceal from their peers. Sequencing months is even harder than days, for there are twelve of them. It no longer astonishes me to find that high school dyslexics cannot necessarily recite the months in order, nor do they know how many days are in any given month. And, not surprisingly, many of them are poor judges of the lapse of time. They miss appointments and are late to class. They cannot judge how much time to allow for getting ready to leave for work. They have difficulty following directions. Once I asked a student to do two things, "Finish writing these sentences and then start reading this story." I came back twenty minutes later to find him reading and the sentences untouched. He was plainly hurt by my annoyance, and I realized the mistake was a genuine reversal. In adult life, these problems may make it difficult for dyslexics to keep certain kinds of jobs.

Many dyslexics have an enhanced sense of the vertical that enables them to excel at certain sports that require balance. Anyone who watched the Olympics probably remembers the dyslexic Greg Louganis poised on the edge of a diving board. Young dyslexics are often skilled at skateboarding, in-line skating, snowboarding, skating, skiing, or horseback riding. One year Shirley Kokesh invested in a couple of unicycles for the elementary program, and within a few weeks, all the students were riding them. At Kildonan we offer horseback riding—in part because of my early love of horses—but also because it is a balance sport, and many of our students take to it naturally, and, of course, it is a great confidence builder. After John List left us as a student, he went on to compete in horseback riding at the state level in Louisiana. For the same reasons, we have always skied in the winter—again, a sport that I enjoyed for many years. Our students are quick to learn skiing, as well as the snowboarding that many of them now prefer.

When it comes to team sports, some are better than others. Baseball requires the fine hand-eye coordination that many dyslexics simply cannot master, much as they would like to please the fond father who is willing to spend time pitching to them. Once, we hired a new sports coach, who evidently failed to listen to my advice when he was assigned to coaching the nine- and ten-year olds. He came to me quite angry and said that one of the students had bitten another child. I asked him what he had been doing with them, and he said, "I was just teaching them to bat." Evidently the level of frustration had been such as to cause one boy to lose control.

We have found success with lacrosse and have played it ever since our last year on the Pennsylvania campus. Soccer and basketball work for us. Some of our students become tennis enthusiasts. Football is less of an option—as one student said to me, "Just try explaining to the coach that you reversed the play!"

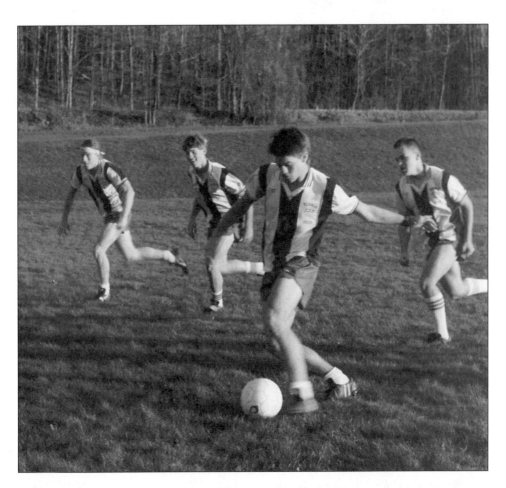

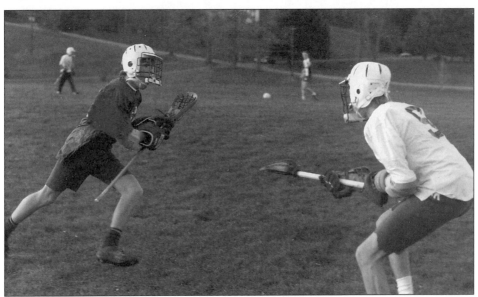

~ 9 ~

Charm

Dyslexic students possess keen powers of observation. They notice things and are entranced by their visual world. The very first thing that attracts the attention of a baby—as we all know—is faces. From babyhood on, dyslexics learn to read body language. They know when a person is pleased, happy, depressed, irritated, or attentive. As teachers, we become acutely aware of this ability. In class, a student answers a question, and though we think we are listening impassively, the student catches a slight shift of expression and changes the answer in mid-sentence. I used to suffer from migraine headaches, and students would notice something about my behavior and ask, "Are you getting a headache?" long before any of my colleagues would notice whatever subtle signals I was giving off.

Sometimes parents or teachers say, "He's such a little con artist." I then try to explain that charm is a god-given gift, an asset, and one that will stand the child in good stead throughout life. Sometimes teachers, especially, would feel that the charm had developed as a compensatory and, they even thought, manipulative mechanism. But I never believed this to be the case. The charm of the dyslexic derives from the keen powers of observation with which their minds are gifted.

Both the innate charm and the powers of observation have many implications for their futures. Obviously, if you are charming, you are going to be popular. Kildonan is a small school, but nonetheless, after students leave us and move on to college, many of them are elected into positions of leadership. They become presidents of their fraternities—as was my nephew, Anthony Poole. My dyslexic niece, Rafaella Bennin, spent her sophomore year at Vassar as a dorm advisor. Sometimes, like Bill Green, they are given a lot of responsibility at an early age; at 23 he was put in charge of a large car dealership, and managed it successfully until he moved on to learning to race cars, rather than selling them. It is no accident that such dyslexics as Charles Schwab and Henry Winkler have risen to lead huge companies. Many of them are successful in starting and running their own small businesses, and, it goes without saying, they are effective in selling their products or services. Melissa Rankin developed a flourishing business in indoor landscaping, and Richard Berg was able to impress important people with his confidence and capabilities in the demolition business. Both of them were former students of mine.

On the national scale, dyslexics are liable to rise to the top in positions of leadership. Winston Churchill's dyslexia has been well documented. From an early age he had difficulty with English skills and, especially, with the Latin then required. He possessed other talents that are typical of the dyslexic: innate charm, skill in watercolor painting, and the ability to visualize the activities of an entire army. Even during the war years he played with toy soldiers, recreating battle scenes and blowing his cigar to create cannon smoke. He had determination in adversity—another characteristic to be addressed in a later chapter. The British royal family certainly appears to have a dyslexic gene. I have already mentioned George VI's stutter. Quite accidentally, I ran into a teacher who had tutored Prince Charles when he attended Timbertop School in Australia, and he commented to me on the extent of the prince's dyslexia. Some members of the current Swedish royal family are dyslexic.

In our own country, Nelson Rockefeller never did learn to read. Even as an adult, he had to rely on memorization. His daughter said to me once, worried about her own son, "Daddy never did learn to read." I have often thought that the forefathers of the Rockefellers and other families built up their fortunes as a result of a dyslexic trait. Woodrow Wilson is said to have been dyslexic. Jack Kennedy was dyslexic, as was his son John—who was hyperactive as well, and had trouble staying in school. Robert Kennedy's children attended The Potomac School, where I taught for many years. As they entered the lower school, they all needed help with learning to read, and, when they came into the upper school, most of them had problems with French and Latin, as well as with the spelling of English.

The Bush family is open in acknowledging their dyslexia, and, of course, it is a source of endless merriment to their political adversaries. While I suspect some of the jokes as being apocryphal, many such as the reversal tendency, the confusion between similar words, and the difficulty in remembering names—especially of foreign countries and their leaders—ring true. One benefit of George W. Bush's dyslexia is the interest he has taken in improving the performance of schools throughout the country. Since, in the past, many prominent families regarded dyslexia as something of a private shame to be concealed as much as possible, the willingness of a family to acknowledge it is refreshing.

Besides innate charm, many dyslexics possess the ability to imitate people. Dunnabeck and Kildonan students can often do devastating imitations of their teachers. Drama is often an excellent outlet for their talents. At the end of the summer program, whenever we put on our final talent show, I am often astounded by what even the youngest ones can do on stage. Susan Hampshire, the British actress who starred in *Upstairs Downstairs* as well as in *Born Free*, is perhaps a classic example. Her delightful book, *Susan's Story*, is still in print. Even as an adult she continued to have difficulty with left/right discrimination. In filming "Born Free," she describes an incident in which she was being filmed running around with the lioness, Elsa.

"I heard 'Action', and suddenly I was chasing Elsa through the long grass.

'Susan, keep running, she's coming round on your right. Run to your right.'

My right—of course. I veered to the left, and ran straight into the lioness.

'Keep going, Susan, run faster. Hedge her in on the left. Bring her into shot. On the LEFT, Susan, LEFT.'

Left, right, right, left—how could I tell the difference? After that little romp I wrote a great 'R' on my right palm and an 'L' on my left and kept them there till the end of the shooting."

A couple of years ago I had lunch with Eileen Simpson, author of *Reversals, A personal account of victory over dyslexia*. She had learned that she was dyslexic, not from a psychologist, but from the poet John Berryman, who later became her husband. She explained that unless she was wearing a ring, she could never be sure about right/left. Actors Tom Cruise and Cher, as well as Jay Leno, have acknowledged their dyslexia.

I once ran across a teacher who told me she pretended to say the pledge of allegiance, and knew that the hand she placed over her heart had to be her right one. When driving with dyslexics, one must be sure to point and say, "Do you mean this left/right?" Once, many years ago, I was tutoring a little Spanish girl. She suddenly became angry and frustrated and shouted at me, "Which /b/ you want? The /b/ that goes this way, or the /b/ that goes that way?" I understood her frustration.

Many aspects of medicine depend on keen powers of observation. There is no doubt that, if they can get through medical school, dyslexics make wonderful physicians. For one thing, diagnosis in part does depend on keen observation, and surgery is often both an ambidextrous task and one that depends on the ability to work in three dimensions. My mother, a sculptor, once gave lessons to a dentist, and subsequently remarked to me, "I think dentistry is a kind of sculpture." The eminent surgeon Harvey Cushing was dyslexic, as was one of the Mayo brothers. The latter was unable to learn enough German to be able to read medical journals in that language. Once I read a biography in which he expressed his anger to his secretary, who was complaining about his spelling.

I used to collect stories about neurosurgeons. One of my favorites is that of a physician who, exhausted by a long day of surgery, commented to his wife on the drive home, "That was a very peculiar speed limit we just passed, 53 miles an hour."

It may have been Dick Masland who advised me, "If you want to find the right neurosurgeon for a critical operation, ask him if he had difficulty learning to read and spell. If he says he never had problems with either, look elsewhere."

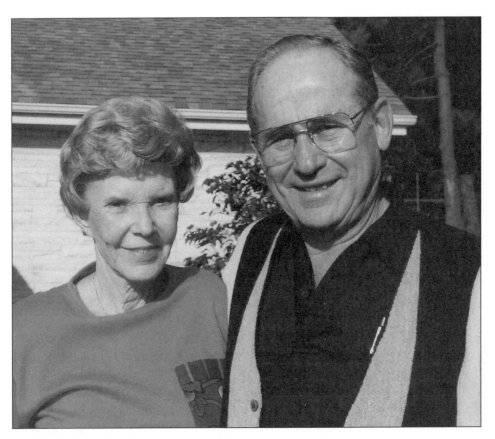

Joan and Kurt Goldman, parents and Board members.

~ 10 ~

❧ Parents ❧

As a young teacher I was always intimidated by parents, nervous about addressing them, and secretly resentful that they seemed unable to understand the struggles of their children. As the years have gone by, I have come to realize just how difficult and painful it is for parents to have a child who cannot succeed in school.

The underlying anxiety of many parents is for the future. They ask such questions as, "When will he learn to spell?" "When will her reading comprehension improve?" "When will he become a faster reader?" "How can I get her to be less forgetful?" "What if he continues this bouncing his knee into adult life when he is at an important board meeting?" "When will she learn to add without counting on her fingers?" For some of these questions, the answer is "maybe later" or "maybe never." And, even better, "it probably won't matter."

Dyslexic fathers often believe that because they made it through school and on to a successful life, their children, especially their sons, should be able to cope on their own, without all this expensive special help. But the world has changed, and more is expected of this generation. I once had a conversation with an apparently concerned father whose son was particularly disorganized in managing homework assignments. I asked him if he couldn't help his son—after all, as a lawyer, he certainly possessed the skills. I was stunned by his reply, "What do you want—my left kidney?"

Sometimes the ambitions of parents lead them to want something for their children that is away from their natural bent. I once tutored a sixteen-year-old who was gifted artistically. He ornamented his essays with little pencil sketches that I thought showed incredible talent. But his father, whose main occupation was managing his investments, had different ambitions for his son and envisioned a business career. He was horrified at my suggestion of an art school. Many years later, the son had become an alcoholic who was supporting himself as a stonemason. I always wondered what his life would have been had he gone to art school. Jackie Onassis did not allow her son John to follow his wish to become an actor—something for which he had some talent—but threatened to disinherit him if he made such a career choice.

I have known marriages that fall apart because husband and wife are split by differences as to what is best for a child. Dad may be set in the role of demanding more than what a child can do, while Mom becomes fiercely protective of that child's need for intervention and support. It is she, often alone, who will go to a school day after day and fight the professionals who may be insisting that their son or daughter is lazy, unmotivated, careless, undisciplined, or just a "late bloomer."

Many parents feel guilty about their early neglect of their child's problem, or even of their abuse—for many of them do indeed believe the professionals who assure them that their child is just lazy, or needs more discipline at home. Not surprisingly, they fall into the trap of putting increased pressure on a child who is already doing the very best he/she can. Sometimes they may even assuage their feeling by complaining about aspects of a program in which they have enrolled their child.

On some occasions, when there is no help available for a child, a parent can be the child's only hope for learning to read and write. As he did with Helaine Durbrow, Dr. Orton guided many parents in the teaching of their children. For families who have no money for tutoring, cannot possibly afford private school, or live in remote parts of the country, this may be the only option. Now that many mothers work, it is more difficult for them to find the necessary time. If a mother is intelligent, has at least a good high school education, and is motivated—as many of them are—she can often be taught to tutor. On a number of occasions, I have recommended to a mother that she arrange to send her child late to school and spend that first hour or so of the day in teaching him herself. Every month or so, she can bring him to me, or consult with me, and I tell her what to do next.

Schools are never happy with such an arrangement. Some of them call me and angrily remark that they are the qualified professionals—not the parent. In response, I have tried to explain that in the three, four, or even five years in which they have had charge of the child's education, they have succeeded only in destroying his self-esteem without teaching him to read or write. Parents who have followed this course of action have always achieved fine results and, in many instances, enabled their child to compete successfully in a regular classroom. I do not, however, believe that such an arrangement is likely to work for older students, who are less willing to be taught by their parents and who need more advanced skills and a higher degree of expertise. My dream would be to organize parents to teach beginning skills so that there would be one on almost every block. They would then tutor one another's children. Students who have never been damaged or destroyed by failure are usually easy to work with. It takes relatively little effort to get a first- or second-grader reading. But by adolescence the years of failure have taken their toll, and the task is far more difficult.

I continue to be amazed—although by now I shouldn't be—at the amount of misinformation, useless cures, and over-generalized treatments that are available, and continue to trick parents into wasting time and valuable resources. Just this past week I worked with a bright little boy whose mother had tried every possible diet, as well as fish oil, colored lenses, eye exercises, balance beams, and shaping letters out of clay. All, of course, to no avail.

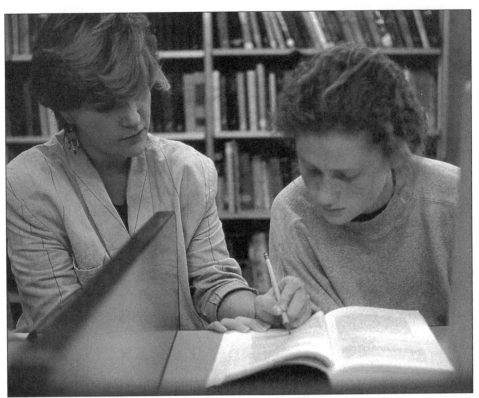

Theresa Collins, who now heads the Language Training Department, tutors a student.

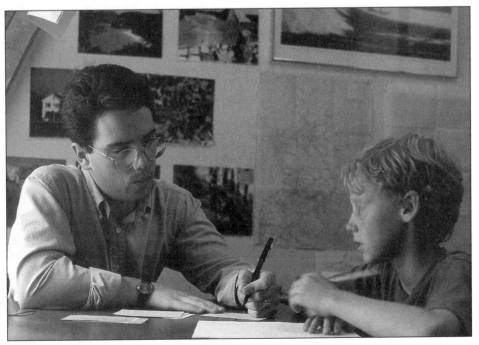

Tutor Joe Ruggiero works with a child.

~ *11* ~

Teaching

One of the reasons why I could never succeed as an administrator is that my real love has always been teaching.

Ever since I started with my "Kippers" at Ruzawi School, teaching has been the thing I love doing above all else. And the one-on-one tutorial is even better. The world vanishes; suddenly there is just me and my student. I have been told, and have noticed this on tapes, that my voice changes when I am tutoring. I think somehow I am activating a different part of my brain—it would be interesting to see whether this is actually the case, and I think the science exists to prove it. Time stands still. I once asked a surgeon what he did during a long operation—did he take coffee breaks, or what? He replied that he was quite unaware of the passage of time when he worked in the operating room. At present I tutor six students in a row with only a twenty-minute recess. At the end of my day I am always surprised to find that this is my last student. Never do I find myself thinking, "two more to go."

My entire focus is on the student—and this is true no matter what their age. I instinctively and effortlessly change my manner to be appropriate for the student. Young children require a teacher to be more energetic and playful than do older students. The output of energy is the same, but it is on a different plane. As students enter my room, I look at them attentively in an effort to assess their mood and state of mind. I greet them warmly, as if they were the first and only student I had ever seen. Depending on what I observe, I begin to plan the lesson. Will we start with oral reading, which we do at some point every day, or with writing? If we decide to write, will we begin with a review of spelling rules and generalizations, or, in the case of an essay or a paragraph, with a discussion of what it would be fun to write about? I never make a detailed lesson plan, although I may jot down in my plan book a quick note as to something I need to teach in the near future.

As we begin to work, my attention remains focused on my student.

When he or she makes a mistake, or cannot recall something I was sure I had taught thoroughly, my question is always as to why, and what could I try to do differently. As I once learned, we need more ways of explaining than the child has of not understanding. I take advantage of the keen powers of observation of the dyslexic to use gesture, expression, or body language to indicate an error. When the student is reading, I keep the place with a pencil, and simply point when a word is misread or omitted. If a student gives an incorrect response, I may simply shift my position slightly. Silence is useful; often if we wait, a student will think again and come up with a correct response. Some dyslexics process language slowly, and need a little extra time. I tend to encourage students not by saying, "excellent," "wonderful," "good job," etc., but by body language; sometimes I just smile and nod. After all, for a high school student to be spelling a third-grade-level word correctly is hardly "excellent." I never write such comments on the paper of a student, nor do I believe in stickers or other rewards. Carl Kline, the eminent Vancouver psychiatrist and dyslexia specialist, once told me he thought rewarding students for learning was humiliating them. So much for "operant conditioning."

Dyslexic students do not necessarily tell when they don't understand something. This failure to ask is not just reluctance to expose their ignorance in this one-on-one setting; in fact, they often do not themselves know what they don't know. The process of filling the gaps in their knowledge is one of endless discovery. Recently I was working with an eighteen-year old who had been a virtual non-reader. In the course of a single lesson, I discovered that he had no idea what the letters B.C. meant following a date. Then we read a passage in which the bones of Arabian horses were described as "dense as ivory." On a hunch, I asked him if he knew what ivory was. "Poison ivy?" he asked.

My expectations for my students are always high. To expect less than their best efforts is to make them feel that since we don't expect much, they cannot be worth much. Thus, low expectations undermine their sense of self-worth. I once tutored a senior, who came to me with a reputation for never doing any work in the study halls to which she was assigned. One day she walked into my tutoring room and blithely reeled off a list of excuses. I told her that I had better things to do than waste my time with her, and left the room. Never again did she come without her work done. Later, after she left for college, she told a friend that, angry as she had been at the time, the incident was a turning point in her life.

Often we do not find out until years later what a difference the programs at Dunnnabeck or Kildonan have made in the lives of children. It may be only through a chance meeting with a parent or with a former student that one learns the results of one's work. In any event, many dyslexic students have difficulty expressing themselves in words, and they generally avoid writing. However, recently I tutored a girl, Sydney, for a year-and-a-half. She had dropped out of school, and spent a year feeling hopeless and depressed. With her permission, I am here reproducing the unusually eloquent letter she sent me after starting college.

> *"As I sit here and attempt to write a note to the most influential woman in my life, I find myself at a loss for words. What you have done for me is nothing less than miraculous. The confidence I have gained, as well as the skills you have ingrained in me will carry me well beyond college and far into the future. I wish I could express my gratitude in words. However, none seem to fit. Your friendship has helped me through the most difficult transition in my life. I now know that there is nothing that I can't do. I love you and respect you more than you will ever know. Without you I could not be me. For everything that you have done and all that I will do I want to thank you."*

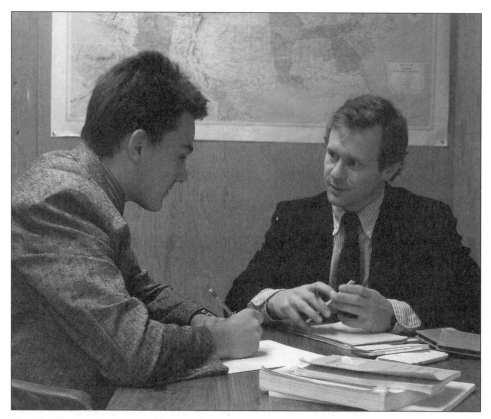

Eric Hill tutoring a student.

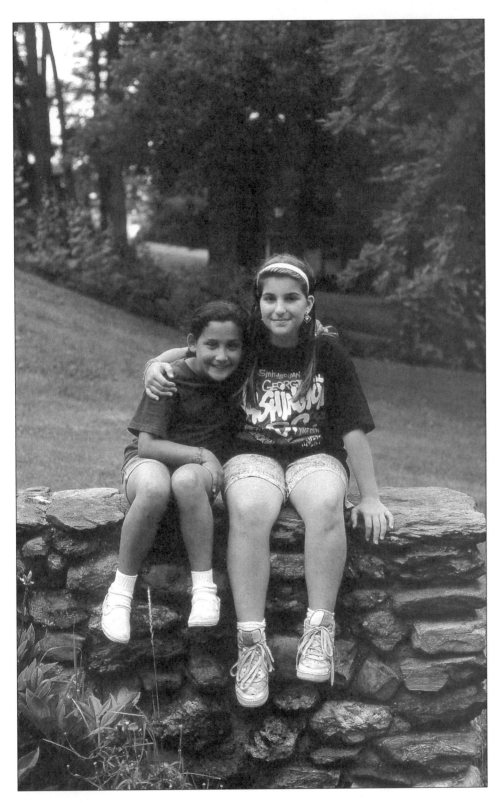

~ 12 ~

To Tell or Not to Tell

The dilemma used to be, and for many still is, do you admit to your dyslexia? Whom do you tell, and how?

Bill Green told me about his desire to keep his dyslexia a secret, against the advice of his father:

"When I applied to college, my father had insisted that I tell the colleges that I had dyslexia. And I did so at certain colleges, but at a lot I didn't. The problem I had was that as soon as somebody knew that you had dyslexia, they wanted to help you, and if you didn't take their help, a lot of times people were offended. I generally wanted to work things out on my own."

K.P. Augustine, another former student, shared Bill Green's feeling that sharing information about his dyslexia would not result in his getting the kind of help he needed.

"I've only leveled with a couple of teachers. When I first went to Frostburg, I had a really good advisor who told me to go up to every teacher and tell him I was dyslexic. I got the impression that teachers would help you, but they would also treat you differently. Also, the help they offered was not always what I wanted. For instance, I was given taped books, but I didn't find them helpful because it was hard for me to listen to the tape and read my text at the same time and I'd have to go over something two or three times and keep rewinding the tape recorder."

Colin Poole, my artist nephew, reflected on the effect that disclosing his dyslexia might have not only on his teachers, but also on his peers.

"Now I tell people I am dyslexic, but throughout school, I didn't want to. In college I would talk to teachers before tests and say, 'I'm dyslexic. I'm not sure if you understand what that means.' They'd say, 'Of course I know,' but usually their concepts of it were way off base, 'You

read backwards.' Even my peers had misconceptions. Once I spoke to a girl in a gym. She's known me for a long time and I told her. She pointed to the exit sign and said, 'What does that say?' Occasionally teachers would say, 'Well, tell you what, we'll give you an extra hour on this test.' I didn't want it. I wanted to be treated like everybody else. Besides, an extra hour wouldn't have made any difference; if I was going to fail the test, with an extra hour I'd still fail, and I knew it."

Colin devised his own study techniques: he cut up his texts and made them into posters, and, incidentally, made the honors list every year.

Melissa Heliker, one of the first girls in the Kildonan program, reported similar difficulties in getting the right kind of help.

"At Chico State I introduced myself to their handicapped department and met some individuals who were involved with dyslexia. I went to one or two tutoring sessions but never went back. Their approach was that it was O.K. not to read everything, and their way of going through a text was to blank out certain words and make sure you comprehended everything regardless of whether you read the words or not. I didn't feel this was a proper approach."

Sometimes, it is easier to lie.

Then there is the problem of what to tell a prospective employer. Paul Barbeau said,

"Last summer I worked in the land title office. I shouldn't tell you this, but they asked me if I was dyslexic, and I said no because I was desperate for the job, as I needed the money to finance my education."

K.P. Augustine said,

"Sometimes people ask me if I'm dyslexic, and I won't come right out and tell them I am. I don't want any kind of special treatment, and I don't want too many people to know. I've known a lot of people who are dyslexic and they'll tell everybody, and when they do something stupid people will say, 'Ah, that's because he's dyslexic.' People have this preconception, 'If he does something stupid, it's because he's dyslexic and not because it's his personality.' Sometimes I have told people, and they have said they never would have guessed it. Personally, I don't think it is a stigma, but a lot of people think you can't do something if you are dyslexic."

Dyslexia can be an embarrassment that continues on beyond college and into adult life.

At age 30 Brian was a successful chef, but he said:
"I still don't write and I don't even like to think about it because I like to communicate so much and I just can't. I dictate a lot. For instance, I'm too ashamed to put my handwriting up in the kitchen. So I'll just dictate the worksheets or I'll write them out and somebody who can decipher my writing copies it."

I received a call from Wayne, who was at that time working as a truck driver in Texas. He came up for a promotion that would involve doing some writing and had panicked. I advised him to go and talk to his boss about his spelling problem. His boss told him to take a pack of 3x5 cards and write the words he needed for reference. He added, "I never knew anyone who could spell who was any good at driving trucks." You can imagine Wayne's relief.

Some years ago I received a call from a woman who had been referred to me by her psychiatrist. As head of a large Catholic school, she often had to send hand-written thank-you notes to parents and others. Her inability to spell was a source of profound embarrassment, and she wondered whether it could be corrected. I spent a couple of hours working with her. In the course of our conversations, she explained that she had gotten through both high school and college by cheating, and I thought what this must have cost her—a devout Roman Catholic—in terms of guilt and shame. As well as giving her a spelling test, I administered parts of the high-school level of the *Slingerland*, those that involve visual recall of complex shapes and of groups of letters and words. She missed virtually every single item on the latter. I explained to her that, while there were certainly tutors who would take her money—she lived in New York— her spelling could never become good enough to be dependable. I advised her to buy some beautiful cards to send as thank-you notes, so that writing could be kept to a minimum. She could then have her secretary, or a friend, write out some all-purpose sentences for her to copy. Competent and successful as she was, somewhere in the back of her mind must have lurked the suspicion that being a bad speller meant being a bad person.

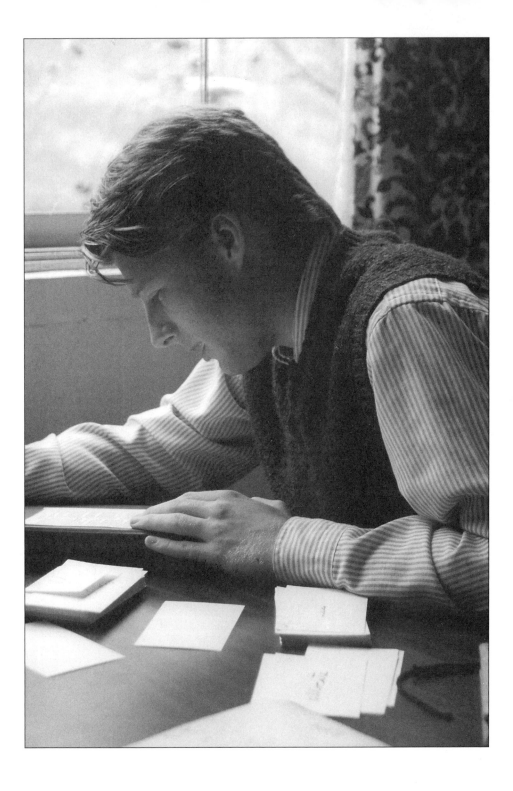

~ *13* ~

❧ *Do You Read?* ❧

For most dyslexic students, learning to read is the turning point in their lives. Some of them become avid readers, often developing areas of passionate interest. A fifteen-year-old student of mine, Kyle Morrissey, is fascinated by the Civil War, in which several of his ancestors fought. While he still had great difficulty decoding most texts, he could flawlessly read the names of all the great generals and battlefields. At Ruzawi School, a seven-year-old boy in my class practically taught himself to read because he enjoyed *Dr. Doolittle* so much. One summer I taught a little girl who was determined to read every last one of the Narnia books. Harry Potter books are relatively difficult, yet sufficiently engrossing that students with relatively weak reading skills persist in their efforts. At least three of my former students have read their way through law school; moreover, I know of five who only learned to read in their late teens and who have gone on to get Ph.D's in various subjects. On the other hand, knowing how to read does not necessarily mean developing a reading habit.

Some dyslexics have been so hurt by their school failure that they never want to have anything to do with books. Benjamin Siff explained it this way: "*Most of the reading I do is in technical publications. Reading… it's like eating a bad hot dog when you are a child, and you don't eat it again. It's a painful experience.*" He added, "*The woman I used to go with never understood why I didn't read. She graduated from Yale and reads a lot. She learned about the world by reading. I learned about the world by seeing and doing.*"

On the other hand, Johnny Hoover enjoyed reading and did a lot of reading at night. He said:

"*I read all my old college books; I didn't get anything out of them then, but now I can. When I am traveling I usually carry one of my old literature books and read the short stories in them, because I know I can pick it out now, but I couldn't pick it out when I was in college. I got all these paperback books and they are great. I read a book, and I then want to get the hardback copy, the nice big one, because I am proud of that book and I want it to stick with me for a while.*"

Like Henry Winkler, dyslexic actor who played "The Fonz" in "Happy Days," Joe Vickers has a library of all the books he has ever read. He says, *"I even stole books from school; if I read it, it went home to Charlotte. I love short stories, about twenty-five pages. I read it, get it, and go on to the next one."*

Colin Poole started reading when his father got him a subscription to *Time*. He said: "Maybe it's made for dyslexics. A lot of the articles are very short. You don't have to read a chapter; there isn't a chapter there. A lot of the articles are just a single paragraph, or two or three paragraphs joined together."

After a while, *Time* magazine got pushed aside, and during his meals he'd sit down with a book. He told me, "This summer I've read about eighteen books. They are all lined up on my shelf, and I have them inset a little bit so I can say, 'From here to here I've read.' And probably by the end of the year I will have read many more books than I have read in my entire lifetime." Interestingly enough, he had a sense that the skill might not last, "There are times when I think this is just a fluke, I'm going to snap back fairly soon, and I'm not going to be able to read any of this, and it is going to be back to ten pages an hour." Then, a few years later, Colin discovered talking books. As he works in his studio, he plays them. He showed me the library list of available books, about fifteen pages in length. He had checked off the books he had read, more than half of them.

Colin's sense that the skill so painfully acquired might be lost reminds me of a story Angie Wilkins tells me about her grandson. She and her husband had established a tradition of taking each grandchild when he turned ten on a special trip of the child's choosing. Her grandson was dyslexic and had just finished with Jemicy School, where he had learned to read. For his birthday trip, he had chosen to be taken to Montreal to watch the Rangers play. After arriving at the hotel, the three of them sat on the couch; Angie and her husband read the paper, and, at the child's request, handed him the sports section. After a few moments, Angie noticed tears running down his cheeks, then he got up abruptly and went off to another chair. Soon sobs were wracking his body. Angie got up and sat beside him to find out what the trouble was. He was heartbroken because he had lost the ability to read—he thought that was because he had left the school where he had learned. Of course he couldn't read—the paper was in French.

~ 14 ~

Training Teachers

For a long time teachers were trained in an apprenticeship model. Anna Gillingham had teachers watch her work and then assigned them to teach a single, carefully selected student. After a while, they would be assigned a second student, whose needs were somewhat different. I learned from Helaine Durbrow in much the same way during the summers I spent at her camp in Vermont. The kind of instruction that works best is diagnostic-prescriptive. The tutor observes the student constantly, notes the areas of difficulty, paying careful attention to errors, and then devises appropriate teaching strategies. Always, the teacher needs more ways of explaining the material than the child has of not understanding it.

While the Gillingham program has a carefully structured beginning sequence, it is not a cookbook. Pacing is crucial: Anna Gillingham used to say, "Go as fast as you can and as slow as you must." A number of methodologies have evolved that attempt to lay out a program in such a way that the teacher can work through the sequence by simply turning the page. While some of these are certainly better than nothing, they cannot replace teacher training.

When I started Dunnabeck, tutors came a week to ten days early for a period of intensive training. Because the group was small and collegial, tutors learned from one another, and were able to share problems and get advice from the more experienced staff throughout the summer. Later, we increased the tutor-training period to two weeks, both before the camp program and at the beginning of the school year.

Tutoring involves a sound knowledge of the phonology and structure of the English language—complex, as it is composed of Anglo-Saxon or Germanic as well as Latin and Greek elements. Our most successful trainees were usually English majors, and, if they had some background in a foreign language, preferably Latin, so much the better. While there are certainly exceptions, we learned to avoid hiring Special Education teachers from the public schools, as they were usually too set in their ways to learn a new approach; once they began working with students, they were prone to revert to doing what they had been taught previously. Moreover, their training does, of necessity, equip them to deal with a wide variety of disabilities, without concentrating on any one in depth. Also, they were deeply sympathetic to their students and afraid of being too demanding.

Unfortunately, it takes a tutor at least three years to become truly proficient and able to work with students of any age. During the training period, it is often difficult to predict who will become proficient. Sometimes teachers will be outstanding during the training period, quick to master the phonology and procedures. But then, when we watch them working with a child, we are disappointed. On the other hand, others who have little background, and have difficulty with every aspect of the training, go on to become outstanding tutors. While I have trained some men who have become excellent tutors, in general it is a skill that women seem to acquire more readily—perhaps because they are more prone to have the necessary patience to go through the daily routines.

Not only tutors, who work one-on-one with students, but also classroom teachers who are to work with dyslexics, need to be trained. They have to know enough about the language so that they can help students cope with subject-matter vocabulary by breaking words into syllables and teaching the more important meaningful parts, or morphemes. Knowledge of common Latin prefixes and roots and of Greek elements — especially useful in the sciences—makes all the difference. Properly equipped, a teacher can help students decode unfamiliar words and learn the requisite vocabulary. Moreover, to work successfully in the classroom teachers have to be sensitive to individual differences. They must be able to engage students who may be non-verbal, and willing to give all students sufficient time to process and respond to questions. They must know how to devise multi-sensory methods of imparting information. Multi-sensory does not just mean showing videos, but engaging the student in thinking, in speaking, and in creating. Above all, these teachers have to have some understanding of the sort of confusions and mistakes to which the dyslexic mind is prone.

Dyslexics often have particular difficulty with names and with new vocabulary. When I read a book with a student, we may be into the last chapter before the student can infallibly read the name of the protagonist correctly. Once I tutored a high school student from the competitive St. Alban's in Washington. I asked him how he thought he had fared on a recent important history test. He replied, "Either I aced it or I failed it." He went on to explain that the test had involved an essay comparing the political philosophies of Jefferson and Madison. He knew the material well, but was afraid that he had reversed the names. Indeed he had, and he failed the test. Another time I was teaching algebra to a group of fifteen- and sixteen-year-olds. We had spent some time discussing exponents, and then went on to an exercise that involved reading them (e.g., y squared, x cubed, b to the fifth). When it was Keith's turn he said, "x cute" and, as I waited, "No, that's not right. I mean x quote." Keith was bright and good at math, but auditory input was a problem for him, as it is for so many of these students. At the end of every term, when I worked with students doing individual testing, I asked a number of the younger ones what they were learning in history. On one occasion, the first said they were study- ing "this person who defeated the big ships by sailing around them in smaller ships," but was unable to recall the name. The second one thought his name was St. Francis of Assisi. The third one got it right, "Sir Francis Drake."

In 1995 a group of us established the Academy of Orton-Gillingham Practitioners and Educators under the aegis of the New York State Board of Regents. Concerned that there were no standards for training, and that parents had no way of determining whether or not a tutor they hired was properly qualified, we set about establishing the much-needed criteria for certification. Then we went on to the accreditation of training programs and schools that delivered appropriate services. As schools and training sites strove to meet the standards required for being recognized by the Academy, the quality of the teaching improved. Kildonan, Dunnabeck, and our training institute, KTI, have all been accredited.

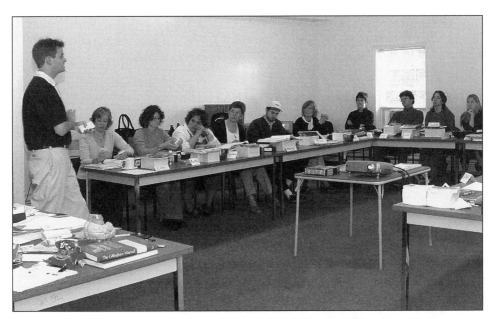

William Van Cleave works with an Associate Level Orton-Gillingham Course.

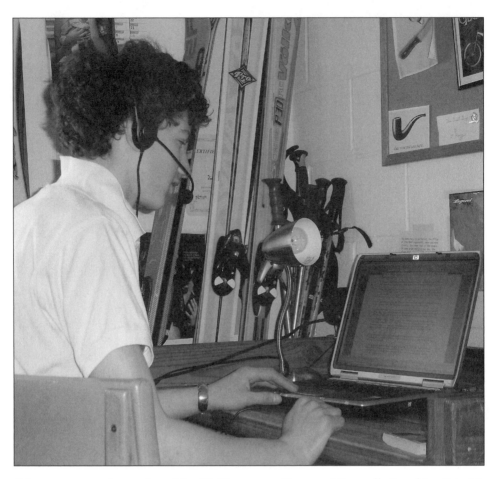

My current tutoring student, Tim Hollinger, uses Dragon NaturallySpeaking® *in his room in Goldman Hall.*

~ 15 ~

Coping with College

It is important to remember that the transition from high school to college is challenging for any student. For instance, in high school students spend most of their academic time in classes, with only two or three hours per night of independent work required to succeed. In college students may spend only two to three hours a day in classes, but are expected to devote four to six hours a day to independent work. Self-discipline and time management are crucial skills for success in college.

Dyslexic students may need an extra year, or more, in order to finish a degree. They need extraordinary determination. They must have the ability to discover their most successful avenues for learning, and to devise study techniques that capitalize on those. Finally, they need to select a course of study that capitalizes on their innate talents.

K.P.'s remarks reflect his determination:

"I guess I am a little more determined than a lot of people. I am amazed at people who drop classes the first or second week of school. I usually wait until I know I can't do it or I'll stick it out. I always wait until the very last day to withdraw. Sometimes if I stick it out, I end up getting a bad grade. I don't know if it is because I'm dyslexic, or if it is just my nature, but if I really want to do something, I'll do it no matter what. I don't second-guess myself. I always think, 'What if I stuck it out just a little longer?'"

Colin spent his first all-nighter working on a paper, confident of a good grade, only to have his efforts rewarded with an F. After that, he never picked up another paper—if he failed it, he didn't want to see it.

For a student like Johnny Hoover to have coped with college required tremendous effort, as well as a support program. He must have been eighteen before he learned to read. I worked with him over the course of two summers. Fortunately, his college offered a good support program with a variety of accommodations. He has gone on to a successful career in business.

Because of his dyslexia, Bill Green had not fared too well in high school. He said, "I think one of the main reasons I went to college was strictly to show my teachers, parents, and everybody else that I could do it. People didn't think I was college material, and I just wanted to show them, 'Hey, if I put my mind to it, I can do whatever I want.'" His first year there he got A's in everything he took. Having achieved his original goal, he became bored and did less well the following year.

Melissa organized study groups and put information on cards. Colin cut up the art history book, and created posters by pasting pictures of artists and their work on large sheets of paper.

Selecting the right program is ultimately crucial, and determines whether or not a dyslexic student can finish college. In general, dyslexic students do best in a small college, where their teachers get to know them outside the classroom and can appreciate their many talents; moreover, a small school is likely to afford greater opportunities for the leadership and the athletics in which dyslexic students often excel. Small classes, or even a tutorial program—such as that experienced by Paul Barbeau at Hull—are suited to the learning style of the dyslexic who has difficulty attending to lectures.

Because of the federal laws, all colleges must provide a bare minimum of accommodations for any student with a documented learning disability. But for students with dyslexia, it is important to find a program that offers the right level and type of services. Some colleges offer note-taking services, which alleviate the difficulty the dyslexic has in simultaneously attending and taking notes. Some colleges even offer tutorial services of various kinds. While peer tutoring can be useful in helping with content or with mathematics, only a skilled professional can improve writing skills.

Colin Poole selected Connecticut College for its strong arts program. The first class he attended was Philosophy 101, which he found painfully difficult. During his freshman year he took an introductory course in anthropology, taught by a teacher he thought was great. He had gone to college with a firm notion that he was not going to become an art major, because artists starve—a price he was not willing to pay. While he continued to take art courses on the side, after that first course, he declared his major in anthropology. But then the anthropology courses became more theoretical and dry, and the last semester of his senior year, he became an art major.

Melissa Heliker enrolled as a biology major in Cal Poly, San Luis Obispo. She found the school extremely difficult, as she was competing with pre-med, pre-vet, and pre-dental students. Together with her future husband, she then transferred to Chico State in Northern California. He was in the agriculture department majoring in Ornamental Horticulture. As she put it, "He came home enjoying his classes, and I came home upset about lab work. He took field trips, and I never had field trips. All his friends were a lot of fun, and mine were dull. And so I changed my major. I took Ornamental Horticulture, and I loved it."

Paul Barbeau, a Canadian, discovered that he could get a law degree in England without first having to complete four years of undergraduate study. He enrolled in the University of Hull in northern England. There was some cultural shock: "With 180 of us there were four showers." He thought, "There is no way I can live here—I have to shower every morning." But he needn't have worried; he usually had the showers to himself! He felt that the great thing about the English university was the tutorial system. He had two tutorials a week with six students and one law professor—not a teaching assistant, but an actual professor. He also had about 15 hours of lecture a week, an essay, and reading assignments. The essays were marked but the mark did not go towards the degree. He told me:

"The result was that you felt more comfortable and you would take risks. At U.B.C. (the University of British Columbia) I see some students who are only concerned with doing the absolute minimum to get the 70% or whatever they are interested in getting and don't take a stab at it to do that little extra bit."

For most dyslexics, college is tough. All students find ways of coping with the stress of college life—you have only to think about the activities of fraternities and sororities. But for the dyslexic student, for whom sitting at a desk and studying can be torture, various forms of extra-curricular activities are a necessity. Many of them play sports, but they nearly all need some extra activity.

Here are some stories of how some of them coped.

Kindra, a fashion design major, explained to me that while she found the swimming she loved time-consuming, it energized her so that she was actually able to be more effective when it came to study time. She felt that without sports, she would have frittered the hours away.

Paul Barbeau played a lot of squash, as, while Hull didn't offer much in the way of sports, there were six squash courts. But he spent more time traveling around in England, going to London and visiting museums.

Colin Poole was interested in weight-lifting. During his freshman year he was part of a group that persuaded the school to use the funds from video games to sponsor a little weight room. He managed it with a friend for two years, and after he graduated, he managed it alone. His senior year he had a full-time job working for a health management organization. That same year he was also House President of his dorm. He also managed to keep animals, despite the college ban on anything but fish. His sophomore year he kept a little boa constrictor. Colin loved birds and had always kept them throughout his school years; he had pheasants, ducks, pigeons, partridges, and quails. His freshman year, he had two doves. His senior year he built a box attached to the outside wall of the dormitory and painted it to match the color of the outside wall so people wouldn't see it. He kept four pigeons in it, until someone noticed what he was doing! Against all expectations, Colin made the Dean's List every semester after his first, despite huge handicaps. Perhaps what saved him were the birds, the gym, and the huge snake.

John Breeding enjoyed water skiing and downhill skiing whenever possible. He also had a motorcycle that he rode through the fields and woods and he enjoyed shooting skeet. As well as skiing, Clem Lottimer took up music; he got to know a radio disc jockey from nearby Nashua, New Hampshire. During his freshman year he became a regular, known for spinning Southern rock and blues. Jim Mosca played in a band while he was in school, earning two or three hundred dollars a week just playing for weddings and other events.

James Agenbroad developed an interest in history, and began a hobby that was to extend beyond his college years.

"While I was at college, I joined a medieval organization called the Markland Medieval Mercenary Militia. Markland is what the Vikings called the land beyond Vineland, meaning 'land of woods.' Originally it was a campus organization at the University of Maryland called U. Maryland Medieval Militia, but they had all those people who graduated so they couldn't call it a campus organization, so they created a new one which included the campus and also some other groups, a kind of federation. I did some work with the Longship Company; they have a 32' Viking ship."

He showed me a photograph of the ship, and I was impressed by its size and evident authenticity. Later he worked at the Library of Congress, but his interest in history remained. He was up at Gettysburg as one of the soldiers when they did the re-enactment of the battle for the 121st anniversary. He told me, "There were 15,000 participants doing that sort of thing, so it was a lot of fun, even though we were running around wearing wool in the middle of June."

Because dyslexics often have superior social skills, they frequently find themselves selected or elected to positions of leadership and responsibility. K.P. became treasurer of his fraternity—the largest at Frostburg—and was later elected President. During his freshman year, Jesse Austell organized a group of students to take at-risk youths camping out on weekends. His efforts resulted in Earthworks, which involved fifteen students and five different city organizations. Furthermore, funding will continue to be available for his brainchild after he leaves college.

Sometimes the activities become so engrossing that they usurp the time that should be devoted to academic work, causing parents to worry that their offspring are not studying harder; and indeed, they often do experience difficulty with time management. However, for the dyslexic these activities are the essential ingredient that enables them to keep their sanity as they struggle with academia. Moreover, the benefits derived from those activities can be considerable, in that they often empower students to develop skills and interests that lead to their vocation.

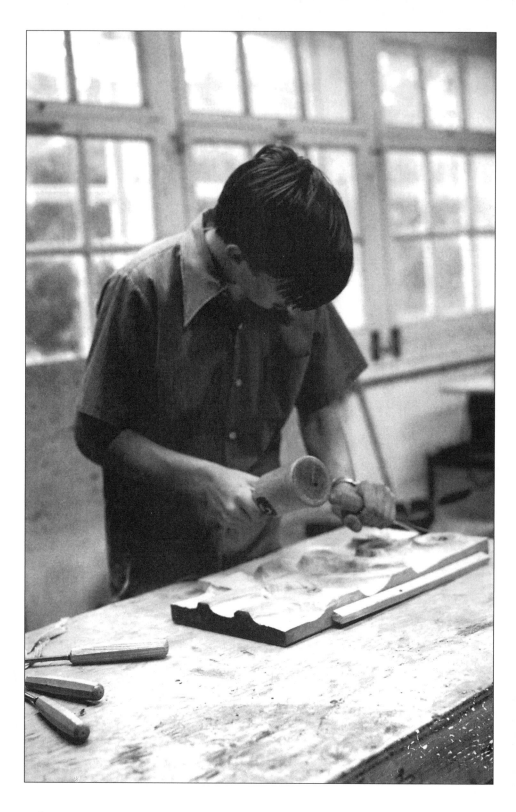

~ 16 ~

Alternatives

While it may seem in American society today that just a bachelor's degree is not enough to secure the career or salary needed for "success," we must remember that there are many who have not attended traditional college programs, but who nevertheless go on to be successful in their own right, and have gone on to lead happy and fulfilled lives. In the past few years we have occasionally had graduating seniors at Kildonan who were with us for upwards of five or six years. It seemed that while they had learned to read, write, and master the content of their classes, school remained an arduous task. Why should we expect them to agree to five or six more years of academic life?

Not all successful dyslexic students start, let alone finish, college, or, in some cases, even graduate from high school. The reasons for that decision are manifold, but most often they find happier outlets for their talents.

My dyslexic South African cousins never even graduated from high school. Yvonne went on to a career in nursing. She went on to work at Guy's Hospital in London as an assistant in the operating rooms. When surgeons had a difficult operation to perform, she was reportedly the nurse they requested. Apparently, the instrument they wanted would be in their hand before they even asked. Ashley studied photography with a famous London portrait photographer, before he returned to Natal and eventually took over his father's farm. Farming, with its many-faceted demands, is the kind of occupation suited to the talents of the dyslexic mind. Incidentally, he became a skilled polo player, and played on the Natal team that competed with the British team, which included Prince Charles. Polo is a sport that enables dyslexics to capitalize on their enhanced sense of balance.

David Kuypers attended Kildonan, and should probably have stayed on longer. In the eleventh grade he attempted a correspondence course, but didn't manage to complete it. He then transferred to public school and, despite his efforts to keep up with everything, was unable to cope, although he enjoyed the sports—especially the rowing. For a while he worked with his father. They grew kiwi in huge greenhouses—another aspect of farming. Later in life he went on to become highly successful in nursery work, and eventually traveled the country as sales representative of a large commercial nursery, where he put his innate charm to good use.

Some other Kildonan students did manage to finish high school and went on to vocational training, or started working immediately.

School was difficult for John Breeding, but his father had made some careful plans. I remember his explaining to me that rather than subjecting him to Junior college, or local community college, either of which would have involved further struggles with academic frustration and the concomitant loss of confidence, he wanted John to acquire a marketable skill as soon as possible, and start working and earning money. Accordingly, he enrolled him in a one-year drafting school in Baltimore that offered a job-placement service. The last time I heard from him he had secured a job as a draftsman in an architect's office.

Jason Puddifoot was the only one of his graduating class not to go on to college. He said, "I don't really regret not going to university. Academically, I wish I had had a more rounded education, but that can always be corrected." And indeed, he went on to develop a fascinating avocation photographing underwater scenes and wildlife in Alaska.

Jeff Melnyk was failing English 12 by Christmas of his Senior year, but managed to enroll in night school and pass the course. He had taken a lot of metal work, and realized that was what he wanted to do. He found a job opening as an apprentice machinist in a manufacturing company. The day after he got out of school, he started work and has worked ever since. He went back to the British Columbia Institute of Technology for five weeks of every year to earn a machinist's ticket, a tool-and-die ticket, and a mold-maker's ticket. His studies involved a lot of algebra, and in anything he does at his job, he uses both algebra and trigonometry.

Some dyslexics find academic work a struggle—in part because of their reading difficulties, but also, I think, because school continues to be emotionally associated with their early failures. Once they achieve success in their jobs, they are unlikely to go back to school, even though they could probably do so successfully.

Lee Dance, who went on to work as an auctioneer, stopped college after a semester-and-a-half. He said: "I wish I had finished. I like what I'm doing, but I also know that I need to take more courses, and eventually I'm going to. I've taken a couple of courses in business and I did okay. But I still have trouble wanting to go to school."

Sometimes the reason for dropping out of college was that the courses seemed irrelevant to the job experiences they had already had. Bill Patterson had studied cooking in France and loved it, but when he enrolled in Cornell he struggled with food chemistry and felt, "Who cares about the molecular structure of lemon juice and milk?" He concluded that he could better use his time working in the industry, and got a job as a chef.

Bill Green studied engineering but quickly got bored with the curriculum. He said:

"It was too easy for me and a lot of the things that you have to study don't apply to real-world situations. After all, I had been working in the construction field since I was fourteen or fifteen, even before I could drive. Then, that summer, after my first year of college, I had worked as a civil engineer doing survey and layout work building the harbor tunnel. Back at school, we started to solve the same problems over and over again and I started to lose interest."

Sometimes an interest developed in high school leads into a career, as the following story illustrates.

Lee Shryock started building stage sets while he was in high school, and then got a scholarship in stagecraft at the local community college. He ended up with a degree in carpentry technology and went on to a successful career in building construction.

Brian Siff attempted college for two or three terms. One of his courses, called *War in the Classical Tradition*, revolved around books ranging from *The Iliad* and *The Odyssey* to *The Thin Red Line*. He said, "It was all long novels, and of course I hate to read. I didn't read all the books, but I read enough to get an A." In high school he had started a tree business with one chain saw and some telephone climbing spikes. He said:

"I remember being up there and getting cramps and seizing up; it was sometimes scary and always difficult. My thinking was that this would get me to study, that this would be my inspiration for going to college. But as it turned out I just became more and more enchanted with work, and grew to enjoy physical labor and the thinking that's involved with taking trees down. I loved the complicated physical task, which is for me, an art form."

Nowadays, colleges offer support programs and accommodations— untimed or extended testing time, books on tape or CD, note-taking services, and even scribes. Computer software such as *Via Voice* or *Dragon NaturallySpeaking*® enables students to dictate their ideas straight into written form. As I write this page, I have a student who acquired the new version 8 of *Dragon NaturallySpeaking®* just last weekend. He spent half an hour training the program, and yesterday, Thursday, he dictated a five-paragraph essay that was virtually flawless. This story may sound like an anomaly to those who have used earlier versions of the program, and often needed to train the program for extended periods of time. The *Kurtz-Weil* and other machines scan texts. Computers are becoming increasingly sophisticated and equipped with not only spell checkers, but also grammar checking systems. But when our first students went off to college in the seventies and eighties there was little help available.

I heard various stories from students that reflect the lack of understanding of some of their college teachers. K.P. Augustine had a teacher who didn't care what his students wrote, as long as it was grammatically correct. He told him, "If you can't write, you can't think." Another student approached a professor and tried to explain his difficulty with spelling, only to be told, "There is a dictionary. Use it." The problem with this advice is that dyslexic students never know which words they need to check; moreover, if you have no idea how to spell a word, it is difficult to look it up. One of my students tried to approach a professor with an explanation of dyslexia, only to be told, "If you have that problem, you don't belong in college."

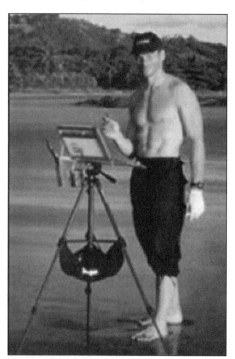 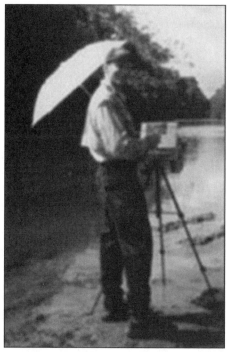

My nephew, Colin Poole, at work. You can view more of his work at colinpoole.com.

~ *17* ~

The Year 2005

The year 2005 marks the fiftieth year of Dunnabeck and the thirty-fifth anniversary of Kildonan. Of course, there have been thousands of changes in the years that have intervened since the founding of the two programs.

Ronald Wilson, our headmaster of nineteen years, has had the creativity, the wisdom, and the foresight to lead the school forward, to make sure it does not stagnate, and to implement the changes necessary to keep the school viable. Educational administration has become immensely complex. Nowadays, changing contemporary standards of what is politically correct, and layers of regulations and laws, require skill to navigate. It's a long way from the simpler days when we started the school.

We have been blessed with wonderful trustees. Kurt Goldman—our founding trustee and for many years my main support, guiding me, encouraging me, and reining in my dreams when they exceeded the bounds of reality—continues on our Board. Both he and Eli Hoffman, who joined the board while we were still in Pennsylvania, have continued to contribute generously not only financial support, but time and advice, and have inspired others to join them. Dr. Thomas J. Emmen, whose son, T.J., was first tutored by my daughter Sheila many years ago, is still on our Board. Kurt's daughter, Debbie DiBianca, joined us recently. Richard Berg, whom I tutored when he was a student here, replaced devoted and generous Leisket Mills, who chaired the board until her death in 1998. Even though he has moved to Florida, where he runs a highly successful business, he makes frequent trips to the school and never misses a board meeting.

Our population of students has continued to grow and now numbers just under 150. They are guided by a faculty of about sixty and supported by an administrative staff of ten. The complexities of legal and regulatory demands have added dimensions to educational administration and financial management quite undreamed of in the days when we had a

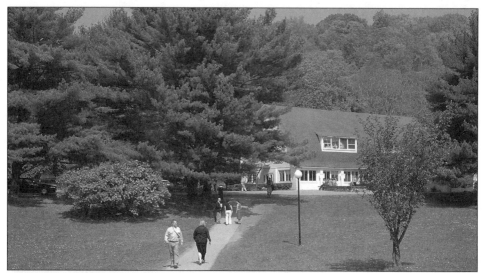

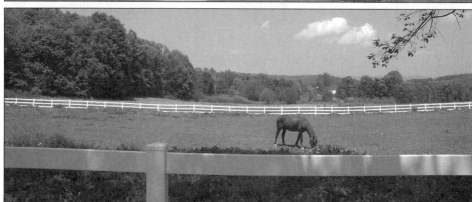

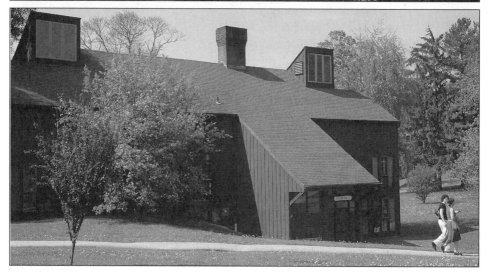

Our beautiful campus! To see more photos of Dunnabeck and Kildonan today, click on our website: www.kildonan.org

124

single administrator—albeit an extraordinary one, Renata Hermes. When we moved the campus from Pennsylvania, we were fortunate to find a marvelous business manager in Ann Still. As well as our headmaster, today we have an academic dean, a dean of students, and an assistant head. The assistant head, William Van Cleave, also conducts much of our teacher training, runs our outreach program, lectures and trains teachers in nearby public schools, and speaks at major conferences such as those of the International Dyslexia Association. Our academic dean, Dr. Robert Lane, besides supervising curricula, testifies at hearings when parents need an expert witness in order to secure funding for their child. Ron Wilson has organized the faculty who supervise the residential program into three teams, each headed by a "crew chief." Since the teams rotate, the burden of residential duties does not fall too heavily on any one individual or group.

Some years ago, we added an elementary program for grades one through six. We became fully co-educational, although we still have fewer girls than boys. While research suggests that dyslexia is equally distributed between male and female, my own experience indicates otherwise. Our population shifted, and now most of our students come from contiguous states and from New York City. In part, this shift is the result of the growing awareness of dyslexia, and of the many local day programs that offer, or purport to offer, services. In order to adapt to this situation, Ron Wilson began admitting day students, and instituted a five-day boarding program. Some students now leave on Friday afternoon and return on Sunday evening. While five-day boarding would appear to offer students the best of both worlds, as well as making the program more affordable, it does have some disadvantages.

The Board has always believed that tuition funds should be used for education of our students and not for erecting buildings, and they have assumed responsibility for raising the necessary funds for projects. Thanks to their generosity, we have been able to add several buildings. The Elementary School building is named for Shirley Kokesh, and incorporates the Learning Center named for Leisket Mills. We have built two modern, fireproof dormitories to replace the old wooden buildings: one for boys, Goldman Hall, and a girls' dormitory, named for me, to accommodate our growing population of girls. Many of the former buildings have been renovated. We are still hoping to build a new dining hall within the next few years. At of the time of writing, the Board has committed the necessary funds to replace the Maintenance Building—in a sad state of disrepair—and to start work on the gymnasium. We would love to be able to add an indoor riding ring and a swimming pool, but since these cost an estimated $250,000 and $100,000 to $300,000 (depending on whether we build an outdoor or indoor pool) respectively, they'll probably stay on the wish list for a while, until some inspired donor provides them.

While my original plan was to have students stay for two or three years, and then, as their skills improved, to move on to other schools, either public or independent, many parents want their children to stay for longer. Some remain with us until they graduate. This change has necessitated the development of a more formal curriculum, in accordance with New York State mandates. Each of the four departments—mathematics, literature, social studies, and science—has a department chair to plan curricula and supervise the teachers within the department. Dyslexic students need multi-sensory instruction, not just in tutorials but also in their subject matter classes. They cannot be expected to sit still and absorb information through lectures, but must be kept engaged and actively involved.

The most important department, as it is our *raison d'etre*, remains Language Training. When I left the school for a few years—first to take care of my mother, then to train teachers in the public schools and to write and lecture—Shirley Kokesh succeeded me. She did a wonderful job, first of working with Language Training, then working as director of education, and finally with running the elementary program, where she developed a remarkably innovative math program. Her legacy in the latter lingers on, and students often surprise visitors by saying that math is their favorite subject! We were heartbroken when Shirley left to take care of her aging father and stepmother. Long-time tutor Laurie Cuddy took over the Language Training department for almost a decade, and not only trained the teachers but also ran Dunnabeck after Penny Crawford and Nick Edgerton left. At present, Theresa Collins does the important job of making sure we follow the guidelines established by the Academy of Orton-Gillingham Practitioners and Educators. Not only does she train teachers, but supports and shepherds them through the challenging task of learning the craft of tutoring.

After Shirley Kokesh left, Francie Borden and Sandy Charlap took over as co-directors of the elementary program. They have extended the art program, added a music program, and developed a Parents' Association, which has been wonderfully supportive in raising funds for a number of enrichment activities, such as expensive field trips that are outside the school budget.

Val Imbleau, our wonderful nurse, stayed with us for twenty years, and we still miss her. She cancelled a vacation to nurse my daughter Sheila in her final days, and I am forever grateful. Patrick Lane, who worked with her, was such an incredibly dedicated individual that after his death, we named the Health Center for him.

It is sometimes difficult to persuade teachers and staff members to stay in our rural environment for lengthy periods of time. However, besides those already mentioned, Trish Roberts has been with us for sixteen years and keeps meticulous records as Director of Development. Lisa Lawrence began as a tutor, but moved on to develop expertise in various forms of technological support essential to many of our students—she is now in her eighteenth year at Kildonan. After graduating from Kildonan, Karl Oppenheimer returned to us as a faculty member. He currently serves the school as Assistant Director of Admissions, President of the Alumni Association, and lacrosse and ski coach. Finally, the school would not be able to function without George Murphy, who is in his twenty-second year of working in the maintenance department, which he now heads. His duties are manifold: he keeps the many buildings functioning, plows snow in winter, mows lawns in summer, harvests hay for the horses, yet is never to busy to rescue a faculty member whose car won't start or whose power has gone off.

The sports program has been expanded to include more competitive sports events. We now compete with other schools in basketball as well as in tennis, lacrosse and soccer. Two fine tennis courts, gift of parent and board member Patricia McLaughlin, are in constant use throughout most of the year. Many dyslexic students are talented athletes, and having an appropriate outlet for their skills is of paramount importance.

Aside from the daily one-on-one tutorials, most of the practices established in the early years of the school have continued. We still have a horseback-riding program, although now not all students ride. As of this writing, we still do not have a proper gymnasium; the winters here are cold and the ground often snow-covered, but the ski program saves student morale and helps get us through the winter. During the winter term Thursdays are devoted to skiing, as well as the snowboarding which many students now prefer. In February, the middle and upper school students still spend a week at Killington, Vermont. The art department established in Pennsylvania gained new strength under the leadership of Jen Harmon, and many of our students go on to art schools. We are still a coat-and-tie school, with the innovation of dress-down Wednesdays. One minor change I regret is that faculty members are no longer on a first-name basis with students; because they are all dyslexic, they have difficulty remembering the names of the teachers!

As for me, I am privileged to pursue my love of tutoring at both Kildonan and Dunnabeck, leaving administration and all the complexities of running the school and the camp to others. I continue to marvel that a dream I had so long ago, to educate students one by one, has been embraced by so many. I now feel secure in the knowledge that the school will survive long after I leave the planet, and that it will continue to grow and make a significant contribution to the lives of all who attend—

one by one.

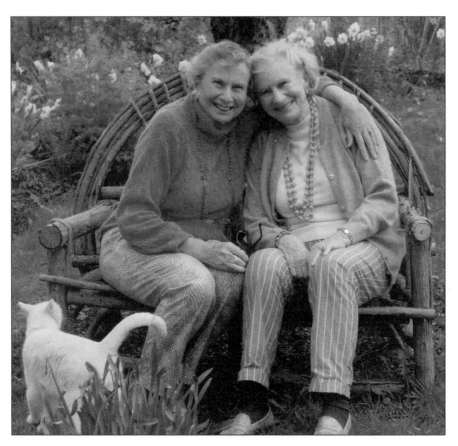

P.S. My sister and I are now the closest of friends!